*More Praise*

# A Maverick of Medicine Speaks to Women

At last, women and health care providers have a champion who is not afraid to step outside of the box and, in frank terms, tell it like it is. The medical system is broken. Pharmaceutical companies and HMOs have turned what was once a noble profession into a business dominated by the bottom line. It's time for the public and the profession to regain control. Reading this important book can be the vital first step in taking charge of our most valuable asset—the health and welfare of our people.

— Rob Robertson, M.D.

Duane Townsend is an extremely talented, well educated and brilliant "maverick." A fantastic book from a fantastic gynecologist.

— William B. Saye, M.D.

Dr. Townsend does a brilliant job of articulating the merits of preventive medicine. It is a triumph for a physician with such impeccable credentials to embrace the life-changing benefits of alternative medicine.

— Cynthia Champion-Olson, N.D., C.N.

Duane Townsend is, as the book title indicates, a maverick by nature. Many of his ideas, initially greeted with skepticism and even outrage, have ultimately proven to be correct. Inside these pages, he presents the case for a variety of unconventional approaches for preventative and therapeutic purposes. An impressive and timely book!

— Malcolm Coppleson, M.D., A.O., F.R.C.O.G., F.R.A.C.O.G.
Former Head of Department of Gynecological Oncology, King George V Hospital,
Royal Prince Alfred Hospital, Sydney, Australia

# A Maverick of Medicine Speaks to Women

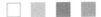

A WORLD-RENOWNED GYNECOLOGIST'S
SOLUTIONS FOR A BETTER WORLD IN
WOMEN'S HEALTH CARE

Duane Townsend, M.D. and
Rita Elkins, M.H.

WOODLAND
PUBLISHING

Library of Congress Cataloging-in-Publication Data

Townsend, Duane E.
   A maverick of medicine speaks to women : a world-renowned gynecologist's solutions for a better world in women's health care /Duane Townsend and Rita Elkins.
      p. cm.
   Includes bibliographical references and index.
   ISBN  1-58054-350-2
   1. Women—Health and hygiene—Popular works. 2. Women—Diseases—Alternative treatment—Popular works. 3. Women's health services—Popular works. I. Elkins, Rita. II. Title.
RA778.T653 2003
613'.04244—dc21

                        2003009467


For information, contact: Woodland Publishing, 448 East  800 North, Orem, Utah 84097

ISBN 1-58054-350-2

Printed in the United States of America
Please visit our website: www.woodlandpublishing.com

*To the thousands of women who have permitted me to
take care of their health problems*

*And to my family—Joan, Eric, Gwyn, Denise, Eryn, Jacquie, Nina,
Lillian, Ed, TG, Calvin Sr., Calvin Jr., and Jeanie*

# Contents

# Preface

A little over two years ago I was chatting with this book's coauthor, Rita Elkins, about the profound health implications of isoflavones and how to make estrogen safe for women. Before I knew it, we were collaborating on a book. "Duane, you have no idea how many women need to hear what you have to say. What's more—you have the credibility to say it. As a seasoned medical professional with a lifetime of experience, publications, honors and most importantly, as a cancer patient yourself, when you speak, people will listen." I told her that the health benefits of a supplement called transfer factor alone should be making the six o'clock news. We also both agreed that when it comes to disease prevention and viable alternative therapies, ignorance still pervades the medical establishment. And after considering the many remarkable stories of my patients (though the book contains only a tiny sampling), we decided to write this book.

Unfortunately, many subjects pertinent to women's health could not be adequately covered in these pages. Consequently, I've created a website that offers a wealth of information for all women and will eventually offer interactive sites. Visit www.askdrtownsend.com for in-depth discussions on women's health issues and the latest on new natural medicines. In addition, there are many fantastic resources listed in the back of this book that can assist you in your quest for improved health.

# Acknowledgments

I would like to express my deep appreciation to all of the teachers, colleagues, friends, family members, co-workers and patients who have enriched my life and shaped my role as a physician.

***Undergraduate Studies at the University of California at Davis:*** Kappa Sigma Fraternity, who took me in as a member and where I met Truman Johnson, M.D., and Jim Truman, M.D., whose advice led me to seek a career in medicine; and the holstein cow that cemented my decision to go into medicine.

**UCLA Medical School:** Horace Magon, Ph.D., and Paul Greenberg, Ph.D., who after my interview accepted me to UCLA Medical School on the spot, for which I am eternally grateful; Baldwin Lamson, M.D., and Roy Wolford, M.D., both in pathology, who exerted tremendous influence in convincing me to stick with my decision to stay in medical school.

**Residency UCLA:** Daniel Morton, M.D., who ran the department and whose tremendous patience was mystifying; John Kelly, M.D., who epitomized the kindness and caring of a true physician, as did Don Hutchinson, M.D., who delivered my first three children; Leo Lagasse, M.D., a fellow resident who played a major role in my decision to enter academic medicine; and William Dignam, M.D., who often quelled my rebellious nature.

**City of Hope:** Ralph Byron, M.D., Robert Yamamoto, M.D., and Dan Rhiiamaki, MD., three outstanding physicians who taught me the best in compassionate care for the cancer patient.

**Faculty UCLA/ Harbor Hospital:** Ted Quilligan, M.D., then chairman, who took a chance on me and gave me the opportunity to seek my own areas of research; Val Davajan, M.D. (deceased), who provided much needed levity during times of stress; Dan Mishell, M.D., currently chairman at USC, whose intensity and tenacity prompted me to publish many of my papers; Don Ostergard, M.D., without whom the colposcopy and cryosurgery projects might never have been completed; Peggy Fiorentino, R.N., a superb research nurse for the cryosurgery project; Joan Nielsen Townsend, R.N.C., N.P., and Maureen Donovon Leyva, R.N., the original "supernurses" of the Porta-Pap Project, and whose energy and enthusiasm led to the hiring of Pat Perkins, L.V.N., and Jacquie Drew, L.V.N., who served as the second tier of "supernurses"; Jeanne Copeland Francis, L.V.N., who was originally a ward clerk and then became a "supernurse" and introduced me to my future secretary at USC, Eleanor Gibson Williams.

**The Porta-Pap Program:** All of the above "supernurses," plus the Pap clinic employees at USC who donated their time to attend the thousands of women who didn't have access to health care.

**Faculty USC Medical School:** Ted Quilligan, M.D., Robert Israel, M.D., and Paul Morrow, M.D., a fellow gynecologic oncologist whose wit and dry humor would surface when we really needed it (he also epitomized the true intellectual physician); Phil DiSaia, M.D., another colleague in gynecologic oncology who went on to become one of the leading oncologists in the country; and to the many oncology fellows at USC who were and still are a credit to the specialty and the school.

*Pap Clinic Employees:* The "bunch" from Harbor, plus Jimmye Mason, L.V.N., Mary Brooks, secretary, Rachael Villasenor, L.V.N., Vicki Reyes of Outreach, and Carolyn Gerscher, R.N.

*The Fellows at USC:* The "Canucks," physicians from Canada who specifically came to USC to study colposcopy and then took the concepts back to Canada; Gordon Lickrish, M.D., Director of the Colposcopy Program at Toronto General Hospital, Toronto; Louis Benedet, M.D., professor and Director of Gynecologic Cancer Program, Province of British Columbia; Michael Roy, M.D., professor and former chairman of the Department of Obstetrics and Gynecology, Levaele University, Quebec; and Amadio "Denny" DePetrillo, M.D., professor and Director of the Cancer Program, Ontario Province.

*The DES Group:* The nurses and secretaries who helped me with the DES project, including Linda White, R.N., Christina Perez de Benest, R.N., Sandra Sanchez, secretary, Linda Kovacs, secretary and manager, Eleanor Marks, medical records specialist and computer consultant, Terri M. Spector, back office assistant and records specialist, Julie London, receptionist, Lynn Utsunomya, back office and records specialist, and Debi Uberman (along with Kathy and Pamela Johnson), our medical records specialist, Tevilla Riddell, back office and records specialist, Mary Tucci, medical record's specialist, and my personal secretary, Eleanor Gibson Williams, who put up with my erratic behavior for ten years, and who eventually literally ran the L.A. County/Woman's Hospital; the "Aussies," physicians from Australia who frequently came to the United States to help teach colposcopy courses and all became close friends; Malcolm Coppleson, M.D., Bruce Dawson, M.D. (deceased), and Ellis Pixley, M.D. (deceased).

*Cedars-Sinai Medical Center, (my first experience with private practice):* Judy Reichman, M.D., with whom I shared office space for eight months, and who is now *the* celebrity doctor; Robert Futoran, M.D., a gynecologic oncologist with whom I worked; and Mac Wade, M.D., Chief of Obstetrics and Gynecology, who broke the rule of a "closed" staff so I could work at Cedars.

*Sacramento, California Private Practice:* Greg Graves, M.D., and Jake Owens M.D., surgical oncologists with whom I worked for over four years, and without question are the finest surgeons and physicians that I've ever known and scrubbed with; Tim Russell, M.D., the most incredible radiotherapist that I've ever known; Fran Sunseri, my personal secretary in private practice; and Jim Harris, M.D., surgeon and senior member of the group who was always exceedingly calm in the heat of "battle."

*Sacramento, UC Davis:* Beverly Kelly, my secretary who had to put up with my ADD; Renae Woolfork, R.N., and Kevin Kaufman, R.N., research specialists who were constantly bombarded with new ideas; Lloyd Smith, M.D., Ph.D, a vegetarian whose eating habits I initially mocked but now admire, and who currently serves as chairman of the Ob/Gyn Department; and Walter Kinney, M.D., board certified in internal medicine and obstetrics/gynecology (one of the brightest physicians I worked with, and who is now recognized as one of the leading researchers in HPV).

*Salt Lake City, Utah, Private Practice:* Gary Johnson, M.D., my former associate who is now deceased; David Quinlan, M.D., whose ideas never ceased; Kim, our back office assistant who taught me a lot about what goes on behind the scenes; Emily in the back office who continued Kim's education; Patti Tabbish, back office nurse who was always thorough and dependable; and Janette Clayton, our current secretary who has to keep track of the thousand of new ideas that I continually come up with.

*The Soy Sisters:* Carolyn Horsley and Kathleen Done, whose lives and superior health have given me an enormous understanding of how lifestyle and diet choices can change our lives for the better.

I also wish to thank my family members for their ever-present support and the countless women who have placed their trust in me. I have been privileged to serve them as a physician and friend.

# Introduction

**I don't mind** being called controversial. You might say I've earned the right. To me, controversy is nothing more than knowledge in the making. For more than forty years , I've run the full gamut in gynecology and witnessed the deterioration of the American health care system. And I'm not afraid to say so. Moreover, because I've made it my business to pay my dues as a physician, I can openly demand a mandate for change.

For you, the women reading this book, the effect of our present-day medical system has been nothing less than devastating. What was once a compassionate profession characterized by caring and qualified physicians has turned into a depersonalized, political empire driven by power and greed and controlled by Corporate America. Unfortunately, you have taken the brunt of this medical mania. You have suffered the abuse of a health care system that has become narrow minded, HMO manipulated and pharmaceutically dominated.

Slow to change and sadly subjugated, physicians need to redefine themselves as true health care providers. How they relate to women's disorders is a great place to start. The rising cost of health care, coupled with indifference to or even disdain for treatments not brokered by pharmaceutical reps or authorized by HMOs, has limited women's choices. In too many cases, the persistent trust women have placed in their primary care providers and gynecologists has been rewarded with confusion and mediocrity.

Scores of women undergo unnecessary surgeries and take untold amounts of minimally effective prescription drugs. In addition, many doctors, because of time constraints imposed by HMOs, often skate lightly over their patients' symptoms or dismiss them altogether as psychological. Doctors, we can't claim ignorance! There is clearly enough available data supporting safe and effective therapies that can significantly reduce the incidence of cancer, cut heart disease in half, decrease Alzheimer's, slow aging, lessen the miseries of PMS, substantially reduce the billions of dollars spent on unnecessary drugs, and squarely tackle the hormonally driven health problems unique to women.

Specific alternative remedies and lifestyle changes need to be recognized as viable treatments. To my colleagues I say, "Physicians, heal thyselves and get with the program!" Complementary medicine is taking hold with or without you. The sooner the medical world learns to emphasize a healthy lifestyle, proper diet and specific natural supplements over prescription medications and surgery, the sooner the absurd costs of health care will dramatically drop. Why? *Because we'll all be healthier!*

Don't get me wrong. I'm no pushover for using every supplement that claims to be "natural." To the contrary, I insist on scientific proof. Just as I may proclaim my opposition to medical practices that should be abolished, I don't hesitate to expose holistic hocus-pocus. In this book, you won't find lengthy lists of supplemental therapies, unproven treatments for women's disorders or lifestyles that are impossible to maintain. What you will find is my belief that eating a certain way, exercising, and using the right nutritional supplements can truly improve your health.

I firmly believe that genetically speaking, we should be living over one hundred years (and healthy years at that). Unfortunately, our dreadful diets, lack of exercise and reliance on pharmaceutical drugs has cheated us out of meaningful longevity and quality of life. For many of us, our senior years are spent with doctors who prescribe enormous amounts of medication, many of which—contrary to what they were designed for—disable us physically and mentally.

As for me, my involvement in alternative medicine has produced a tremendous improvement in my overall health. Before discovering the value of alternative therapies, I had already become a cancer statistic (discussed later in the book). Currently, I am well into the Medicare years and can do things now that were impossible just three or four years ago. I stay up late, take long walks, manage a grueling schedule (in fact I flew over 300,000 miles the last two years without ever becoming sick), and I no longer suffer from indigestion and insomnia. Not bad, huh? And my fifteen-year-old daughter (who was diagnosed with juvenile arthritis at age eleven) has been virtually symptom-free because of a natural immunity-enhancing supplement called transfer factor. My daughter and I are perfect examples of why all of us can benefit from the best that both the conventional and unconventional worlds of healing have to offer.

To say that the medical profession must be revamped is a gross understatement. The ways in which the medical industry supports and polices itself must change. Conversely, you (again, I'm talking to all the women reading this book) must learn to make appropriate demands of your doctors; you must stand up to your HMOs; and, you must become innately suspicious, appropriately cynical and self-confident. Then you will be entitled to make the best choices for yourselves.

I want this book to accomplish two things. First, it should motivate and empower women to raise the bar when it comes to their health care. Second, I hope to spur my colleagues to reevaluate their priorities and not be afraid to challenge HMOs (or insurance companies, or whatever governing body is causing them grief). The revolution is on, and I'm on the front lines. This book is the result of decades of personal experience and research. It is a testament to my own commitment to demystify women's health conditions and their viable treatment options. As corny as it may sound, I consider myself an advocate of women—not only my patients, but also the women who work in my profession. I endorse their causes and acknowledge their complaints.

Last, but not least, this book serves as an indictment against corporate health care, which has transformed what was once a noble profession into a shortsighted financial quagmire. It's a call for an end to the suppressive behavior of HMOs, increasingly shabby medical practices, uncalled-for surgeries, and the misuse of powerful hormonal drugs for women. I challenge my medical colleagues to not only inform themselves about the scientifically documented value of many natural therapies, but ultimately to use them. After all, shouldn't we all want the same thing—to better the health of our patients?

Chapter 1

## My Journey into the World of Women

Men forget everything; women remember everything. That's why men need instant replays in sports. They've already forgotten what happened.

– Rita Rudner

**Whether they were** my patients, my nurses, my colleagues or my family members, women have always played an integral part in my life. In the course of "poking and prodding" them, and after countless consultations, examinations and operations, I have realized that women are nothing less than remarkable creatures. They are sharp, tolerant and able to cope with enormous stress (both physical and emotional). And when it comes to miseries resulting from their "femaleness," I am convinced that their doctors could and should do better.

With that said, you may have noticed the book cover describes me as "world-renowned." While the editors aren't quite lying, you're probably asking yourself "Who is this guy?" The truth is that while I am well-known in medical circles, especially in the areas of gynecology and oncology, I'm not a celebrity doctor who appears on the television morning shows. For that reason, I want to tell you who I am, how I got here, and why you should trust what I have to say. Especially when it comes to women and their health.

## School Daze

In high school, I was an average student, but I did know one thing—that despite my father's love for his profession, engineering was not for me. I decided to become a veterinarian because I liked animals (and still do). Unfortunately, due to my less-than-stellar grades and my inability to focus, few colleges would have me. It wasn't until my adult years that I realized that for most of my childhood, I struggled with ADD (attention deficit disorder), a condition my parents understandably failed to recognize. As it was, this inability to concentrate ended up serving me well. My overactive brain prompted a steady flow of new ideas, many of which would eventually have a positive impact on my life and career.

Before I knew it, I found myself at the University of California at Davis hoping to become a veterinarian. I did well there. I also joined the Kappa-Sigma fraternity, which was one of the single most significant events in my life. Because I had achieved the top grade-point average in the School of Agriculture, two of my Kappa-Sigma buddies urged me to change from veterinary medicine to human medicine—that's right, they said I should become a medical doctor.

The prospect made me reel. I believed that in order to become a physician, one had to amass an enormous amount of knowledge, and that was only achieved by a select few. So I queried my own family practitioner on the subject. "How can you possibly know all there is to know about medicine to take care of your patients?" He answered, "I don't." He confided that he was able to discern normal from abnormal, and when the latter presented itself, he relied on the fact that few diseases kill a person rapidly. In other words, he knew that time was usually on his side. After collecting a detailed history and performing a thorough physical, he would carefully evaluate all factors and usually arrive at the right diagnosis. (As a sidenote, it's sad to see that in the midst of our technology-heavy health care system, a good history and thorough physical have been lost in the fray of sophisticated testing equipment, elegant blood tests, genetic counseling and the like.)

My doctor's candid advice impressed me and gave me new confidence, but I still wasn't sure.

## Veterinary Vaudeville

I guess the real moment of *veritas* came after visiting a veterinarian who specialized in large animals. Our task was to artificially inseminate a Holstein cow (one of the largest dairy cows, standing over 5 feet tall at the shoulders). We went into the barn and found the enormous black and white cow with her head in the feeding bin. Of course, our concerns would place us at the opposite end of the animal.

The vet put on an examining glove, called a gauntlet, which wraps up around the shoulders. I was stunned when he reached his entire arm deep into the rectum to palpate her uterus and insert a very long tube containing the sperm into her vagina. With some difficulty, he accomplished the delivery of the thawed bull sperm, but not without incident. Immediately after the deposit, as if to show her disdain for the whole experience, the cow gave the vet a good, swift quick with her hind leg. After sailing backwards and hitting the ground hard, he came up dripping with cow excrement. It was not a Kodak moment, and I thought to myself—is this really what I want to do for the rest of my life?

## Med School Madness

Switching from pre-vet to pre-med wasn't easy. After carrying enormous class loads to catch up on the credits I needed and working three jobs, I decided to apply to medical school after my sophomore year. I was granted an interview with the UCLA School of Medicine, where I arrived an hour late, sat down and broke into a full sweat. After an hour of questioning, the final query put to me by the doctors was "Why do you want to become a physician?" If you think I came up with some life-changing answer, think again. "I believe it would be fun, and doctors seem to make a decent living." They looked at one another and broke out into large smiles, commenting that mine was the first honest answer they'd heard in a very long time. I thought I had blown it and inquired how the interview had gone. They responded, "We are going to recommend you for admission to medical school." I couldn't believe my ears. I was going to be a doctor!

As you can imagine, medical school was tough—little sleep, horrendous class loads, twenty-pound text books—you know what I'm talking about. And I still felt wet behind the ears, struggling with my self-confidence and often doubting that I had what it took to get through school. I felt I was out of my league, so much so that I took a year off to reassess to my future. But I returned with renewed commitment and strong resolve that I could do it.

Eventually I made it through the endless labs, all-night study marathons and exhausting hospital chores. And by the end, I was on track to discovering which areas of medicine I would specialize in—namely gynecology and oncology.

## Special Deliveries: Paving the Way to Gynecology

Between my junior and senior years of med school, I assisted with a most remarkable thing—the delivery of an infant, and not just one but many. This was one of the most rewarding medical experiences I'd had up to that point (and its mystery and wonder never ceases to amaze me). It's difficult to describe with words, but any doctor, nurse or parent out there who has witnessed a child's birth knows what I'm talking about. I had the opportunity to deliver many infants, and each time was just as miraculous as the first. It just never got old.

An unexpected bonus that I thoroughly enjoyed was seeing (and feeling) the parents' joy. We tried to make the labor/delivery an interactive experience, inviting the fathers to feel the mother's contracting belly and watch the fluctuating heartbeat on the monitor. Sometimes we would even sing to the women in an effort to distract them while in the throes of labor. We were also diligent about apprising the dads of any progress because they weren't allowed in the delivery room in those days (most of our older ob/gyn colleagues ignored the men until the moment of truth, when they dryly announced "Congratulations, it's a girl").

During this time, I worked at Los Angeles County Hospital, caring for women who had serious complications that accompanied their pregnancies. Most of these women came from the poor and urban sections of Los Angeles, and many did not speak English. I also saw first-hand what it was like for these women to face a cancer diagnosis. Because they understood little of what was happening to them, they were afraid. Worse, many who had been diagnosed with cervical cancer did not return for a follow-up visit. I felt terrible for these women, so in an effort to help, I would stop by their homes in hope of convincing them to seek treatment. (I can't tell you how many shabby, poorly-lit, single-room apartments I visited.) Sometimes I was successful in seeing them through surgery, and I made it a point to keep in touch with them post-op. Unfortunately, too often I failed. This experience—despite the tragic circumstances—solidified my love of gynecology and oncology.

## One Unforgettable Experience

There are some patients that you never forget. While a first-year resident at UCLA, I was called to the emergency room at three in the morning to evaluate a young nurse named Paula who had tried to terminate her pregnancy. She was at least twenty weeks along, and in an effort to terminate her pregnancy, had injected a poison called potassium permanganate into her uterus. Most of the liquid had been absorbed by her body, dissolved her blood, and as a result, her kidneys shut down. She quickly went into shock and became comatose. She was close to death for over two weeks.

Then Paula unexpectedly awoke and asked what had happened to her. I explained the situation, and she remembered the events with tremendous guilt. The fetus had died and was spontaneously delivered.

Soon, Paula began experiencing a very high temperature, and a quick examination told us she had an infection in her uterus that was so massive, it was necessary to perform surgery to save her life. When we entered her abdomen, none of her reproductive organs were recognizable. In fact, we had to literally scoop out the organs, which appeared to have been totally destroyed by the infection.

Following surgery, Paula quickly recovered and was sent home. Six months later, after a few follow-up visits, she informed me that her monthly periods had resumed. I told her not to joke about such things. But she was dead serious.

Within a year of her surgery, she married, and since it was obvious she was sterile, I didn't bother to discuss contraceptives with her. But six months later, she missed a period. Miracles weren't in short supply for Paula—her pregnancy test was positive!

Where was the fetus? I was sure there was no uterus. So I told Paula that the pregnancy was dangerous, but she remained unfazed. Finally, at twenty-nine weeks of pregnancy, I convinced her to come into the hospital so that we could closely monitor her. Two weeks later, she suddenly developed severe lower abdominal pain, and we immediately took her to surgery. What remained of her uterus had

---

### Prenatal Progress

☐ ▪ ▪ ▪

During my residency, I was one of the first doctors to do fetal heart rate monitoring. As it turned out, Texas Instruments (then a small company) had developed a device that could detect and record fetal heartbeats. We in turn designed small electrical probes that attached to the infant's scalp while still in the uterus. This allowed us to record the heart rate pattern while mom was in labor.

I was also able to do a limited a fellowship in perinatology focusing on a procedure that allowed us to expose the scalp of the infant while its mother was still in labor, take a sample of blood, check oxygen levels, and so forth. In this way, we could predict whether or not the baby was in any distress, something that is routinely done today. I also participated in a study evaluating the effects of decreased blood flow on sheep fetuses in the womb. It was one of the first forms of fetal surgery. Little did I know that all of these procedures (in one form or anther) would be widely used and become the standard of care today.

---

torn, and her apparently healthy infant occupied her abdominal cavity. We quickly delivered the three-pound baby girl and removed what was left of the ruptured uterus. Paula went home six days later. (And the baby, though born premature, developed nicely. In fact, she eventually grew up to become a nurse.) Medicine is full of miracles and mysteries.

## Freezing: Fast, Safe and Effective

After I completed my residency, I was asked to join the UCLA faculty by an up-and-coming physician named Ted Quilligan. Dr. Quilligan was great—he encouraged real and noteworthy research, and gave us all the freedom we needed. I became increasingly more interested in cancer treatments. So I began exploring the possibilities of using cryosurgery—surgery that uses freezing to remove or treat diseased tissue—as a treatment for conditions of the female reproductive organs. Earlier, during med school, I had seen the value of using cryosurgery to treat conditions such as Parkinson's disease.

So I applied for a federal grant to perform this new technique on female patients. Think about it—if it was practical to freeze difficult-to-reach parts of the brain, getting to the female reproductive organs should be a breeze. The vulva and the vagina could be easily be frozen with no pain. We could even freeze the cervix and have direct access to other areas of the female anatomy with complete safety. For destroying diseased or precancerous tissue, freezing was easier to perform and less invasive when compared to other methods. It was also much better tolerated in terms of post-operative discomfort and pain. The customary procedures—which usually involved heat or scalpels—could cause significant discomfort and were not as efficient as simple freezing.

Although the government was initially apprehensive about my proposal, they would eventually offer me a three-year, $100,000 contract to evaluate cryosurgery of the cervix as a treatment for precancerous lesions. My research helped to open the door to using intra-uterine cryosurgery—something that is commonly performed today.

## My First Female Freeze

I clearly recall the first patient I treated with cryosurgery. Donna had cervicitis, or chronic inflammation of the cervix. I suggested that she have her cervix treated with cryosurgery. Keep in mind that at the time, this technique was found nowhere else, so you might say that I was flying by the seat of my pants. Nevertheless, she agreed to be my first cryosurgery patient.

The surgery went flawlessly—no pain, no real discomfort. However, when Donna returned the next week, she remarked that she was experiencing a heavy watery discharge (what I later figured out to be a normal side effect of cryosurgery). So I examined her and was shocked at how awful her cervix looked. I feared that I had significantly damaged her uterine tissue and may have severely compromised her ability to become pregnant. I had her return for six consecutive weeks, and much to my delight—and relief—her cervix healed spectacularly. Needless to say, I continued the project with renewed enthusiasm, and not much later, Donna married and had two delightful children.

# There Is a Better Way— Cancer and Colposcopy

Ideas are great, but even better is acting on great ideas. Alfred Whitehead once said, "Ideas won't keep. Something must be done about them." During my research with cryosurgery, I reevaluated an old technique called colposcopy (an idea introduced in 1928 by a German doctor but rejected by American physicians). During this time, I talked with one of the worlds' top gynecologists, Dr. Malcolm Coppleson, about the idea of using nurses to perform cervical exams with a colposcope. Dr. Coppleson really opened my eyes to the potential of colposcopy when it came to the early detection of cervical cancer. Using some of his ideas for detection with magnification, I came up with a diagnostic scheme that was published in the *American Journal of Obstetrics and Gynecology*.

I discovered that by adding just a touch of vinegar to the tissue, telling patterns on the cervix are revealed while looking through the colposcope. In fact, the results of our research were so dramatic that abnormal tissue could often be seen with no magnification. Prior to this, if a woman's Pap smear revealed abnormal cells, she only had one option—the removal of her cervix (called *conization*) usually followed by a complete hysterectomy.

Now, by employing the colposcope with the vinegar application, the area in question could be visually analyzed, and if it wasn't cancer, the abnormal tissue could be destroyed using cryosurgery. It was a slick, less invasive procedure and saved enormously on costs. And it could be done in the doctor's office instead of a hospital. More importantly, in cases where only precancerous cells existed, the patient kept her cervix and uterus. (Keep in mind that until that time, millions of women annually had abnormal Pap smears, resulting in untold numbers of unnecessary procedures. With this new process, less than 1 percent were found to actually have cancer and require surgery.) Regardless of all its advantages, it was originally rejected by mainstream medicine. But it would eventually become the gold standard worldwide for diagnosis and treatment of precancerous cervical lesions and remains so today. The approach proved so valuable that we began teaching the techniques to health care providers all over the country and did so for twenty years.

## The City of Hope: Living Up to Its Name

During the course of my residency, I rotated through the female cancer service of a hospital located in Duarte, California. Called the City of Hope, this remarkable cancer center provided free care to those who couldn't afford it. The staff there had a profound effect on my approach to the care of the cancer patient. Their philosophy toward all cancer patients was to keep hope and optimism alive, regardless of their prognosis. They literally creat-

## My Celebrity Pupil

You've probably heard of Dr. Art Ulene, who I trained with at UCLA. He came to work with me at a critical time as we were terribly understaffed. Little did I know that he would become the first and most celebrated doctor of television, also known as "Doctor Feeling Fine!" Dr. Ulene was one of the first to successfully use the media to inform women about breast cancer prevention and detection through self exams.

ed a "city of hope" among the dying and believed that what comes out of a physician's mouth can truly influence the well-being of a seriously ill person. It didn't matter how sick a patient was or how much time they had left, when these doctors met them, their comments were only positive—"You look great today" or "We're going to do everything we can to beat this thing." I learned from them that making life as tolerable and pleasant as possible for the dying was part of my stewardship as a doctor.

Patients have so much to tell us if we just listen. So often, all they need and want is a more personalized touch to the care they receive—something few physicians are good at providing. While my love for obstetrics did not wane, working with these women was equally engaging. My experience at City of Hope led me to eventually specialize in gynecologic oncology, the care of women with cancer of the reproductive organs.

## One Man Among Many Women

Ironically, one of my most memorable patients at the City of Hope was a man. Joe was the only male ever to grace the female cancer ward. I inherited him because he refused to be taken care of by the other two physicians. To say he was difficult was an understatement. However, if you were minus a bladder and rectum and still had cancer that had spread to your bones, all of which caused unending pain, how good would your attitude be? I saw him twice a day, and I was extremely frustrated that there were no medications that could control his pain, not to mention beat his cancer.

One day while driving to the hospital, I had an idea—perhaps giving him some male hormones would perk him up. I wrote the order for the hormone shot that evening, and the next morning when I came in to see him, he was sitting up in bed, pain-free with a huge grin on his face. Before I could say "good morning," he grabbed me by the arm and said, "Doc you won't believe what I dreamed last night!" Apparently his dream took place in a lovely garden full of beautiful, scantily clad women (in fact, he recognized one of them as one of the clinic's nurses who had been particularly kind to him). Well, he began chasing her around with obvious intentions, and just as he was about to reach her, he woke up.

It took him a minute to realize that he was in a hospital. He emphasized over and over to me that his dream was the most incredible adventure he had experienced for some time (despite the apparently disappointing ending). I'm certain that the hormone shot had given him some freedom from his pain and hope that he could live his last days in peace. Though he died a few weeks later, they were the most pleasant he'd had since coming to the City of Hope.

# Nurse Practitioners: Another Radical Idea

During the time I was evaluating the cervical freezing and colposcopy techniques, I received a grant for cervical cancer screening. I hoped that this project would motivate poor women (who had three times the frequency of cervical cancer) to come in for free checkups. Because our budget would not allow me to commission a doctor, I hired two young women fresh out of nursing school. Despite prevailing archaic attitudes about what nurses shouldn't and couldn't be doing, I decided to instruct them in performing pelvic examinations, Pap smears and colposcopies.

As far as I know, this was the first documented instance of using "nurse practitioners" who had been trained by a physician. I believe their experience led to the eventual acceptance of nurse practitioners in medicine and helped stimulate the development of the first training program created by Dr. Don Ostergard at Harbor Hospital (itself another remarkable story). We would eventually be approached by the Los Angeles Regional Family Planning Council to use nurses to administer their services. Since we had the only nurse program in America (and perhaps the world), we received a sizeable amount of money to start it.

## Porta-Pap Clinics

While working at Harbor Hospital, we specifically earmarked funds to provide Pap smears for disadvantaged women. Despite this, they simply weren't showing up at the clinic. We later discovered that many women were unaware of the service because they could not read, and those that could had no way of getting to the clinic. So, with the help of the American Cancer Society, we boldly decided to take the clinic to the women. From this idea emerged the Porta-Pap clinic, which would travel from neighborhood to neighborhood, providing free exams in parish halls, school gyms and the like.

Because male examiners weren't usually too well received by the women, our nurses performed most of the exams. I would only attend to confirm a suspected abnormality. And because there was no grant money allocated for the "portable" aspect of our new clinic, we all pitched in and used our own resources to rent a van. It was the nurses who loaded, drove, and unloaded the van and set up the screening areas. Let me tell you, these were remarkable women in more ways than one. They would work extra hours, create special forms, organize teaching seminars, and do whatever else it took to make sure the projects were completed. (In fact, I thought these women were so great that I ended up later marrying one of them!)

The Porta-Pap clinics were a huge success—they lasted fourteen years and screened over forty thousand women in Southern California, picking up numerous cases of cervical and breast cancer.

## Adele's Cancer: Opening My Eyes

One Thursday, our Porta-Pap clinic was held in a grammar school in Watts. As the evening passed, we picked up several problems, but one in particular stands out. Adele was twenty-six, and this was her first pelvic examination. As I viewed her cervix through the colposcope, it was obvious that she had cancer that was in an early stage. The nurse performed a biopsy, and our suspicions were confirmed. Because Adele was unemployed and without funds, I referred her to UCLA for care since they had money available for cases like hers.

I ended up participating in her surgery (a radical hysterectomy), which was performed by the senior resident under my direction. We removed the uterus and lymph nodes where the cancer might have drained. I made a bet with the senior resident that her lymph nodes would be free of cancer cells since we picked up on the problem so early (thanks to our nurses at the Porta-Pap Clinic). The procedure went well, and Adele had no problems.

Four days after surgery, I received a phone call from the resident—virtually all of her lymph nodes had cancer. The microscopic appearance of her cancer was very unusual, not the typical cervical cancer normally seen in women. Her cancer recurred within a matter of months, and she soon died. I was stunned and became depressed by her death. I couldn't comprehend how a disease could

## Encounters of the Alternative Kind

After working for several years at L.A. County Hospital, I became exposed to "alternative medicine." It started when I heard that some of our cancer patients made regular trips to Mexico to get something called laetrile. Most of these women had exhausted all of their medical options and had little time left. Keep in mind that in those days chemotherapy was only marginally successful. What impressed me was that laetrile (then considered worthless) had somehow worked its way into a medical establishment that vociferously rejected the idea of "alternative" medicine. Yet every time cancer claimed a one of my patients, I came face to face with the limitations of conventional medicine.

To my knowledge, over subsequent years, laetrile has not been shown to have much impact on the treatment of cancer. I have no doubt, however, that future practitioners will consider the ways doctors have treated cancer over the last 50 years as barbaric and overly invasive. And I can guarantee you this—future physicians will look to a broad spectrum of solutions for cancer, regardless of whether they're labeled "natural" or "conventional" or something in between. And teaching their patients to *prevent* disease will be their first priority.

spread so rapidly. Little did I know then that she had a neural crest tumor, a type of cancer that stems from primitive cells occasionally found in the cervix. It is fast moving and typifies the disease at its worst. I had just been baptized into the unpredictable and frightening world of cancer.

# The DES Disaster

As fate would have it, I became privy to one of medical history's greatest tragedies. It was a gross betrayal of the trust patients put in their doctors and in the pharmaceuticals they recommend. This scandal, which first emerged in the early seventies, dealt with the devastating effects of DES (diethylstilbestrol), one of the first synthetic estrogen drugs originally designed to treat menopausal symptoms. Unfortunately, the medical community also touted it as a solution for miscarriages and other pregnancy problems. Consequently, it was widely dispensed to women for several years.

Eventually, a horrible statistic was uncovered—between 60 and 90 percent of daughters born to mothers who had taken DES had abnormal sex organs, and over half suffered from infertility, miscarriages and cancer. The sons of these women also had problems with testicular dysfunction. It didn't take long before DES was banned for use during pregnancy.

The DES tragedy is a sad commentary on the very real dangers of some prescription drugs. In this case, this drug was a threat not only to the women who took the drug, but to their future children as well. Taking DES dramatically increased the vaginal and cervical cancer risk for the daughters of these women. Somewhere between four and six million American and European women, and some ten thousand Australian women, used DES to prevent miscarriage and other complications of pregnancy. Understandably, these women assumed the drug was safe. And as is the case with so many drugs, a long period—nearly twenty years—passed before scientists discovered the dangers of DES.

Assessing the health impact of DES was (and still is) virtually impossible. It became obvious to me that the DES problem was too huge to handle without some outside help. And so along with several others at USC, I applied for a grant to study the daughters of women who had taken DES during their pregnancy. We eventually were able to receive 1.7 million dollars, along with equal funds directed to Baylor Medical School, Harvard Medical School and the Mayo Clinic for this study.

Our mission was to keep tabs on a group of very young women whose mothers had taken DES. Over a period of time, we followed almost four thousand young women who lived in the Southern California area. Once again, we hired several nurse practitioners to assist in examining these young women.

## A Woman's Touch

It came as no surprise that nurse practitioners were more successful in these evaluations than the doctors. As Faith Whittlesey said, "Remember, Ginger Rogers did everything Fred Astaire did, but she did it backwards and in high heels." These exams were given to girls who were between twelve and fourteen years old. You can imagine the anxiety they and their mothers must have felt. After all, the purpose of the study was to determine if they had suffered any ill effects from DES. These youngsters had never undergone any type of female exam, and most of them had not engaged in any sexual activity.

Our nurse practitioners educated these young women prior to their exams, and these kids were just phenomenal. They were so cooperative, and we got to know them extremely well. They became like our own children as we watched them grow into adults. As their confidants, we were privy to the trials and tribulations of their dating years, their marriages and the inevitable problems many of them had in trying to get pregnant. Countless times they would seek our advice about relationships before broaching the subject with their parents. It was a remarkable thing to chronicle the maturation of these young women. The charge of the program was to assess the physical damage of DES on these women, but it became so much more than that.

# Defusing DES Fallout

Mothers who had taken DES had to cope with an enormous amount of guilt. They feared that what they did years ago may cause their daughters to develop cancer. In addition, their children's infertility only served to worsen their feelings of shame. Consequently, we spent hours comforting these moms and their daughters through their ordeals.

Happily, before the project ended, most of these exposed children were able to conceive and carry at least two pregnancies long enough to give birth to healthy children. Just recently, Baylor University examined a number of young women born to women who were exposed in utero to DES. I'm happy to report that these young women have no evidence of the DES damage that their mothers bear.

Although it was a stressful time, the DES experience provided me with tremendous insight on how chemicals can impact not only our lives, but also those of our unborn children. In fact, I personally treated twenty-one young women with cancer due to DES exposure. And while we cured them all, most were rendered sterile before they reached reproductive age.

## The True Meaning of Being a "Complete" Woman

Ruth's case was one I'll never forget. As we sat in my office, we discussed how her mother had taken DES while pregnant. A year before I saw her, Ruth had been given a clean bill of health by her doctor. However, when I closely examined her cervix with the colposcope, I noted a tiny area of red no larger than the point of a pencil that wasn't visible to the naked eye, and removed it. The report showed that it was the type of cancer associated with exposure to DES. After informing Ruth and her mother about the situation, we had a very emotional session and eventually decided that her cancer would respond best to irradiation.

The radiation treatments worked to get rid of the cancer, but the side effects were tragic. She became sterile and began menopause at the young age of twenty-four. And she also suffered extensive side effects that included severe shrinking of her bladder and persistent ulcerations and scarring of her vagina. I saw her and her mother monthly, but my attempts to control her pain and heal her tissue were not very successful.

Still, a year after treatment, Ruth met and eventually married her first husband. Initially he was very supportive, but as she continued to suffer, their marriage became strained. After two years, her pain was gone but the scarring persisted, making sexual relations with her husband impossible. And her bladder was still dramatically shrunken. At this time, I decide to perform a biopsy of the vaginal tissue, and to my utter disappointment, I found that the cancer had returned. Ruth's only option was to have an operation called anterior pelvic exenteration, in which the entire vagina, urinary bladder, uterus and ovaries would be removed. We created an artificial bladder made from her intestines and a new vagina of muscle and skin from her thighs. She adapted well to the changes; however, her husband didn't and soon left her with these parting words, "I want a complete woman."

This remarkable woman would need to have her artificial bladder replaced twice and her vagina reconstructed four times. She also suffered from various other complications. But she never lost hope. If you can believe it, over twenty years later Ruth is physically active and just recently married once again. Moreover, she directs postgraduate programs for physicians and remains one of my closest friends.

## Consider All Treatment Options

Mary, a twenty-six-year-old woman whose mother had taken DES while pregnant with her, was referred to me because of a lump discovered in her vagina. Upon examining her, I told her we needed to biopsy the lump. Mary immediately ordered me to stop the exam, told me where to "stick it" (referring to my instrument), and punctuated all of this by stomping out of the office while uttering a few more expletives.

Later, I convinced Mary to come back for tissue sampling, and the lump did indeed contain the cancer associated with DES exposure. I had to do some fast-talking to convince her that without treatment, she would die. She argued that she didn't want the treatment because it would make her sterile, and she absolutely had to have children.

We finally reached a compromise to treat only the area of the cancer (a little over an inch in diameter) with radium seeds (localized radiation) in an attempt to preserve her fertility. I told Mary that in all likelihood, this would not cure her cancer. But much to my surprise, the lump disappeared and the cancer did not return. About two years later, Mary married and became pregnant. Though happy at the news, I was quite concerned that her baby might be deformed because of the radiation treatment. However, she delivered a healthy seven-pound boy, and two years later had a second healthy child. Both children have grown up without any problems, and Mary has remained disease-free. This experience taught me to never exclude any treatment possibilities.

# Keeping Your Uterus on the Ball

For many years, I firmly believed that women should be given an alternative to a hysterectomy—particularly when they had abnormal bleeding and hormonal drug therapy failed. So, one day in 1998 while mulling over some possible options, I came up with another idea. Why couldn't we roll a tiny electrically charged ball (about the size of a BB) across the uterine lining to destroy it, thereby stopping or dramatically reducing the troublesome bleeding? My curiosity led to the development of the

## The Grass Is Always Greener

I have never hesitated to try a new treatment that could help my patients. For example, while working with cancer patients it didn't take long to note that during their chemotherapy sessions, most people suffered from severe nausea and vomiting, and the drugs used to control these symptoms were often ineffective. During my stay at the Cedars-Sinai Medical Center in Los Angeles, I'd heard that marijuana might be effective for post-chemo nausea. Well, you can probably guess what happened next. After a bit of searching, I found a source of marijuana and instructed my chemo patients to make marijuana brownies or to smoke it prior to and during treatments. Everyone knew when one of my patients was having chemo because the halls of the female cancer service were filled with the sweet smell of marijuana. Let me reiterate here that using marijuana medicinally made a substantial difference for my patients, helping them get through a very difficult treatment.

Keep in mind that several "legitimately approved" drugs are considered controlled substances. Consequently, I saw no reason to exclude a therapy such as marijuana that eases the severe nausea that accompanies cancer treatments. Consider this: According to the Centers for Disease Control and other sources, there are more than 400,000 annual drug deaths from tobacco, 100,000 from alcohol, up to 60,000 from "legal" drugs, and 19,000 from illegal drug overdoses. On the other hand, there have been no confirmed deaths from marijuana. Perhaps we should all reconsider our government's logic when it comes to things like tobacco subsidies and the fight against illegal drugs.

technique, and the procedure did not disappoint, producing excellent results. Soon we began to offer women what we called the "roller-ball" technique, or more technically, endometrial ablation.

After about a year, I felt that gynecologists throughout the country should be offering women this marvelous hysterectomy alternative. So I developed methods to teach physicians the ropes of the roller ball technique, and soon enough the project was taking me all over the country. I really enjoyed observing these doctors at work and frequently held the hands of the patients before and after surgery.

The technique was nothing less than a veritable blessing for women who wanted to avoid the trauma and risk of a hysterectomy, but needed to stop troublesome bleeding. Over the last several years, a number of companies have realized the benefits of endometrial ablation, and other methods of destroying the uterine lining have evolved. People said I was ahead of my time, but I think Einstein put it better, "I have no special talents. I'm only passionately curious."

Of these newer methods, the safest and easiest to learn is cryoablation. A company called American Medical Systems developed a unit to destroy the uterine lining using intense cold. The method is virtually painless and can be performed in a physician's office. Because cryosurgery is so safe, versatile and has such excellent results, I prefer to use it over the original roller-ball technique. Every woman should know that it offers an excellent alternative to hysterectomy. Unfortunately, too many don't.

## The Case of the Off-Color Ovary

Ann was forty-two years old when she came to see me because of an abnormal Pap smear. During her initial examination, I determined that nothing was wrong, and even during a second exam, her colposcopy was clear. I did note, however, that her left ovary was slightly enlarged, which is never really a good sign. I asked her if she was having any discomfort, and she answered no. She did remark, however, that she was receiving hormone shots for weight loss. I suggested that she stop the hormone injections and come back for another exam in eight weeks. She wasn't sold on the idea, but finally agreed to halt the treatment.

When Ann returned her ovary seemed normal, but I still suggested that she have a laparoscopy, a minor procedure where a small telescope is inserted through the belly button and the abdominal contents and pelvic organs can be seen. (Remember that at this time, we didn't have the advantages of CT scan or ultrasound technology.)

Ann strongly objected to the surgery but finally relented. I found that all of her organs appeared normal except for some areas of discoloration on her ovary. So I did a biopsy and sent it to the pathologist before completing the surgery. Something about the whole situation bugged me.

"Well you've done it again," remarked the pathologist when I talked to him. "It's cancer." Though I thought something may be wrong I did not expect that diagnosis. Now what—wake Ann up, tell her she has cancer and that she needs more surgery? Or go on with the surgery and tell her afterward? It was a no-win situation. She would certainly criticize me regardless of what I did. So I proceeded with a hysterectomy, removing both of her ovaries and all the surrounding tissue needed to effectively manage ovarian cancer.

When I informed Ann that we had found cancer and subsequently performed a hysterectomy without her permission, she said, "I thought you might find cancer. I want to thank you for what you did."

Of course, we had Ann undergo chemotherapy. Up to this point in time, virtually all of my ovarian cancer patients had died. She did not. Eventually she became a close friend, and at this writing, is alive and well. For me, her experience brought home the notion that following your intuition is usually a good thing.

## Coming Face-to-Face with Alternative Medicine

Barbara, a recently married woman in her late twenties, sought my help after being diagnosed with cervical cancer. I suggested the usual treatment (radiation) to be followed by a hysterectomy. She responded by giving me the not-so-impressive statistics of such treatments. She finally decided that she would accept surgery but would have nothing to do with radiation. I reluctantly performed only the surgery and then observed—with both incredulity and curiosity—her aggressive treatment of the cancer using an array of methods that I had never heard of, including colonic irrigation and various herbs. (She always called to get my input before beginning a new treatment.)

As it turns out, I operated on Barbara twice more for recurrent cancer, and she eventually died after a fourteen-year battle. I can assure you, however, that if she had followed my original advice, she would have died ten to twelve years earlier. Barbara forced me to consider the notion that her "alternative" treatments must have slowed her cancer.

# Falling into the Loop

During my five-year stint at the University of California Davis, a technique called loop excision became popular for treating precancerous changes of the uterine cervix. The original loops were excessively large and took too much tissue with each treatment, so I developed newer loops that only removed the abnormal tissue. Hence, the acceptance of loop excision accelerated. (Keep in mind that using colposcopy also helped hone in on only the abnormal areas.) Studies confirmed that this technique was superior to other options and is now the treatment of choice for women who have abnormal Pap smears and precancerous lesions of the cervix. I can say with absolute certainty that when well-trained physicians perform this technique, the patient has a 95 percent cure rate for life.

## Seeing the Pitfalls

The cumulative effect of my journey through medicine—and especially my dealings with women—has me convinced that today's health care industry needs a new mission statement. Conventional medical practitioners do not provide their patients with ways to promote and preserve optimal health; to the contrary, they simply "put out fires." Today's medicine is not proactive. Rather, it is reactive, only responding to the onset of disease.

Moreover, many medical practitioners are arrogant, generally unapproachable and have placed themselves on a pedestal (I'll even admit to occasionally having this attitude). If it wasn't taught in medical school or didn't represent the standard way of doing things, it is irrelevant. I often tell my patients that doctors can walk on water, but only when it's frozen.

I rejected the prevailing attitude of the medical establishment, so I had to look into all viable therapies for my patients, regardless of their origin. In addition, as I witnessed the evolution of expensive, high-tech medicine, I watched the demise of doctors who facilitated healing. Patient histories, consultations, carefully formulated treatment plans and follow-up visits have been sacrificed for the HMO business modus operandi. Of equal importance, my own personal experience and that of my patients reiterated the fact that effective alternative remedies are marginalized by most doctors, whose practices leave little time for study. I, on the other hand, have done my homework.

Over the years, I have tried to employ the philosophies of true healing, especially when it comes to disease prevention. On top of this, I've continually searched for better ways to improve the health of my patients, even if I had to venture into uncharted territory or ruffle a few feathers along the way. Keep in mind that once a very prominent British gynecologist/oncologist (now dead) included in his book index this entry regarding my colposcopy procedure: "Colposcopy, the worthlessness of."

Despite the ups and downs of my career in medicine, I wouldn't change a thing. Franklin Roosevelt said something I've always taken to heart. His words were, "It is common sense to take a method and try it; if it fails, admit it frankly and try another. But above all, try something."

☐ ▨ ▧ ▧

# Chapter 2

# HMOs and the Pharmaceutical Empire: Health-Care Heresy

*"They [organized doctors] forget perhaps that medicine is for the people, not for the doctors."*
*– James Means*

**Yes, I am** a product of the mainstream medical establishment. I am also a realist who has come to terms with some basic facts. Let's face it—in the last forty years, the practice of medicine has devolved (to a large degree) into little more than a bureaucratic, drug-dispensing machine fueled by corporate, not patient interests. The old school physician earned the implicit trust of his patients. For women, this was profoundly important. In times past, the doctor's office was considered a sanctum where after careful consultation, the physician integrated the best of all healing options for his patient. Moreover, the personal dignity of the patient was tantamount to respecting the ethics of medicine. So much so, that the doctor/patient relationship was thought of as something sacred. Criticizing these failures, Mahatma Gandhi once said, "I have endeavored to show that there is no real service of humanity in the profession [of medicine] and that it is injurious to mankind."

Certainly we are living longer because of the availability of pharmaceuticals and other advancements. The development of antibiotics alone has eliminated countless deaths. Ironically, however, their overprescription has created a serious new health threat: antibiotic-resistant "super bugs." In fact, the World Health Organization (WHO) has been monitoring this growing danger since 1994 and now believes only global strategy will contain these super bugs.

Likewise, vaccines have reduced deaths from several diseases, but they come with potential risks, including Alzheimer's disease, chronic fatigue, autism, schizophrenia, mental retardation and even death. The controversy associated with giving a series of vaccinations to babies and young children needs further exploration and lucid discussion. Personally, I believe that if doctor's taught mothers to give their children immune boosters before and after vaccinations, risks could be decreased. You see, all immune systems are not created equal at the same age, so side effects differ from child to child. By using certain nutrients, (such as vitamin C, transfer factor, and others) immune reactions can be modified and in some cases, minimized.

Although the mission statement of the pharmaceutical industry is to continue its vigilant quest for health, it sometimes appears as if the last thing it wants is for us to get well. And as long as we don't wise up and change our diets and lifestyles, their business prospects will always look sunny.

Of course, there isn't just one reason for the current failures in health care, but health maintenance organizations (HMOs) and other managed care organizations must shoulder some of the blame. In my more than forty years as a doctor, I've had several run-ins with HMOs and have learned the hard way that too many managed care decisions are based on their bottom line, not on what is best for the patient. Because of HMOs, I have had to operate in unequipped and understaffed hospitals, and I have had to fight to get essential operations covered for my patients. So what happened when I brought these things to the attention of HMO officials? I was dropped from their rolls. I discovered the hard way that when you rock the HMO boat, you get thrown overboard.

I know I'm not the only doctor (or patient) who has had tug-of-wars with insurance providers. I firmly believe that all the red tape, time and money restrictions, and a stubborn refusal to examine preventive and complementary treatments typical of many HMOs has resulted in substandard care for both men and women, and more importantly, unnecessary deaths. Furthermore, the existing bias in women's health care that HMOs—and the medical community as a whole—continue to perpetuate is troubling. The whole system needs to be scrapped if health care is ever going to improve. As long as pharmaceutical companies, HMOs and other for-profit managed care providers are running the show, the focus of medicine will be on the profit and loss sheet—at the expense of your health.

## HMO: Mismanaged Care

With all of the bureaucracy and restrictions associated with "managed care," I think that "mangled care" would be a more accurate description of many HMOs. Their influence has contributed to the lack of progress in many areas of medicine, especially in women's health care, and to overall substandard health care rampant in today's medical system. HMOs have often interfered with what is best for my patients. HMOs have failed to accomplish what they were originally designed to do—control spiraling health care costs. They crashed and burned long ago and what remains is nothing but wreckage. Countless patients and doctors have become disenchanted and disenfranchised by the shortcomings of managed care. The sentiment to exchange HMOs for other programs that permit better exchange between doctors and their patients is mounting.

Conventional medicine has become an industry working under the constraints of HMOs. To make matters worse, HMOs continually refuse to aggressively address the value of sound nutritional practices to prevent the biggest and most expensive killers of our time—heart disease, cancer, stroke and Alzheimer's disease. Furthermore, the "hurry up and treat" philosophy of modern medical practitioners has resulted in harming countless patients and causing countless deaths. According to an article in the *Journal of the American Medical Association,* doctors contribute to 250,000 deaths annually. Personally speaking, the HMO intrusion into my practice boils down to this simple statement—what's best for the patient takes second place to what's economically expedient for the HMO.

## The HMO Way

My first run-in with a major HMO involved a woman named Martha. She had been my patient for over six years and had successfully undergone endometrial ablation. About six months after her husband's employer changed health care providers (for the third time), Martha came in with a serious gynecological condition referred to as a prolapse.

I knew of a new operation that could remedy her problem with minimal surgical time and a more rapid recovery. The only hitch was that the procedure required specialized equipment, and the only hospitals Martha's HMO permitted her to use were not adequately equipped. Their scrub nurses were also not trained to use the equipment. When I complained to the HMO medical director, he told me point blank that I must use the hospitals of their choosing. To help Martha, I tried to be accommodating. I described the operation in detail to the head nurse of an approved hospital and explained what equipment I needed. I was assured that all would run smoothly.

On the day of surgery, things went anything but smoothly. Martha's surgery was delayed nearly two hours because the anes-

# A Brief History of HMOs

□ ■ ■ ■

Managed health care was not always as mismanaged as it is today. In the early nineteenth century, arrangements were made between physicians and groups of individuals to meet their health care needs. For instance, a doctor named Michael Shadid developed a cooperative health plan for rural Oklahoma farmers in the 1920s, where he provided medical care for the farmers for a predetermined fee. And in 1938, similar programs were set up for the workers who built the Grand Coulee Dam, steelworkers, and shipyard workers on the West Coast. Prepaid systems like these served as models for later entities like HMOs. While the original philosophy of these programs may have been well intentioned, what they have evolved into is less noble.

At the end of World War II, a health plan was made available to the public. Then in 1971, the Nixon administration announced a new national strategy with the objective of enrolling 90 percent of the U.S. population in HMOs by 1980. In order to jump-start the program, the federal government established planning grants and loan guarantees for HMOs, hoping to increase the number of HMOs from thirty in 1970 to 1,700 by 1976. Although that goal was not met, there were over six hundred HMOs by 1996 with around sixty-five million customers.

In time, however, enthusiasm for HMOs waned. Why? Because they failed to succeed at their original goal—to control spiraling health care costs. Countless patients and thousands of doctors have become disenchanted and disenfranchised by the shortcomings of managed care. Today, the mounting sentiment is to scrap the HMO format entirely. What we replace it with is hotly debated, but the fact is, HMOs have failed miserably in their original purpose.

thesiologist was "too busy" to start on time. Shortly into the surgery, a vital piece of equipment broke (it was old, but the hospital refused to replace it). Later, when I asked the scrub nurse for the special instruments I needed, she informed me that she had no idea how to use them. The surgery had to be put on hold again so I could teach the nurse how to operate the instruments. All in all, the procedure, which normally takes about sixty minutes, ran about two-and-a-half hours (not including the time wasted by the anesthesiologist).

Post-surgery, I told Martha's husband what had gone on and that I didn't know if I could continue to take care of his wife under the restrictions of his present HMO. About a week later, I received a call from what I refer to as the "hatchet person" of this particular HMO informing me that I was being dropped from their panels. Why? Because I dared to lodge a complaint with Martha's husband. What was even more amazing to me was the fact that they showed virtually no concern for Martha. She saw me for one postoperative visit and then had to start seeing another doctor.

# The HMO Assault on Physicians

Time after time, I've seen HMOs limit the medical options available to my patients. Show me a patient who hasn't had to justify coverage for an emergency room visit or fight to get pretreatment authorization for a needed medical procedure from their insurance provider. For example, I once wrote a prescription for a common birth control pill that is also effective in treating acne. However, because it wasn't approved by my patient's HMO, she was left to choose only from medications that were less potent.

The old-school physician, after a careful consultation, would try to find the best treatment option (not just the best pill) for the patient. He would follow-up with his patients, even doing house calls if necessary. In fact, according to Dr. Harvey Kugel, author of *Talk Medicine,* some physicians are forced to see a new patient *every seven minutes.* Does the phrase "How ridiculous!" come to mind? "I felt like most of my time was spent waiting, and I was shuffled out the door before I had a chance to ask any questions," confided one of my patients about her previous doctor. Another complained that she had to call her former doctor for her biopsy results after waiting a week for him to call her back.

## HMOs Can Be Hazardous to Your Health

The "herd 'em in, herd 'em out" work ethic of today's physician excludes even the most rudimentary aspects of healing. Without enough one-on-one time between doctor and patient, patient histories are often incomplete, and doctors may prescribe treatments without knowing all the facts. Even if your doctor makes time for you and comes up with the best treatment for your health problems, he may still find resistance from your HMO. Managed care providers frequently ration out resources available to doctors such as diagnostic and lab tests, equipment or staff, and they "encourage" their doctors to follow their clinical practice guidelines (CPGs). CPGs limit treatment options to reduce the cost incurred by the HMO and often exclude new, unorthodox or costly tests and treatments as well as brand-name drugs, which in some cases may be more effective than the CPG-authorized recommendations.

If your doctor chooses an unauthorized treatment, he may be reprimanded (or dropped) by the HMO, or you may be refused coverage. In fact, nearly 20 percent of insured women (ages fifty to sixty-four) reported that they did not fill a prescription, skipped a recommended medical test, treatment or follow-up, or failed to visit the doctor at all for a medical problem because of cost, according to the *Commonwealth Fund 1999 Health Care Survey of Adults Ages 50–70.*

# Drugs: The Quick Fix

Benjamin Franklin said, "He's the best physician that knows the worthlessness of the most medicines." In my view, almost every ad that pushes a drug targets a health problem that could be eliminated by a simple change in diet. But which is easier, changing the way you eat or popping a pill? Americans want drugs to fix their depression, conquer their weight problems, lower their blood pressure, and reverse their heart disease, diabetes and sexual dysfunction. What we should be investigating is how we became the way we are.

Two out of three doctor visits result in a prescription, epitomizing the notion "if it ain't broke, fix it till it is." More money is now being spent on prescription drugs than on time spent in the hospital—$500 billion this year alone. For example, when I see a woman who's battling mood swings, weight woes or is concerned about her bones, she is invariably surprised when I recommend that she change the way she eats, begin to exercise, and take nutrition supplements. Why? Because she's used to seeing the old prescription pad whipped out, scratched on, and that's that. Granted, we do have more same-day surgeries thanks to the availability of new endoscopic techniques, and that's a good thing. However, it's estimated that over 150,000 drugs are in use in this country, and scores of new drugs make their debut every year—*are you kidding?* Using drugs has become synonymous with practicing medicine.

Moreover, patients expect to be given pills. Slick and sappy commercial ads for prescription drugs are everywhere and target virtually every age group. You can be sure that there will always be a new drug in search of a market. In the last ten years, pharmaceutical companies have tripled the amount of money spent on advertising prescription drugs directly to potential buyers (us) from $791 million to nearly $2.5 billion. And sales for the fifty most advertised drugs accounted for almost half of the

$20.8 billion increase in drug spending last year. According to the *New York Times,* Merck spent $160.8 million to promote Vioxx, and its sales soared to $1.5 billion last year. This media blitz reduces treating disease to nothing more than a marketing scheme. Furthermore, these ads don't just target prescription drugs. Direct-to-consumer medical advertising is not limited to the pharmaceutical industry. Ads that encourage perfectly healthy people to get CT scans (computed tomography) to detect disease and cancer just jack up the cost of medicine for all of us. A recent report in the *New England Journal of Medicine* pointed out that the inaccuracy or misreading of these tests may cause needless invasive procedures.

## The Truth Comes Out

Six weeks after I had bilateral knee replacement surgery, the physician committee of one HMO met and decided to drop me from their panels. They had heard a rumor that I was retiring (though no one attempted to contact me to verify my plans), so now was a good time to axe me and make it official. They sent my letter of termination to an unoccupied building (one I had long since left), so it wasn't until six months later when one of my patients told me I was no longer on her HMO plan that I put two and two together. My nurse called the HMO and asked what had happened. I was being dropped from their panels because there were enough ob/gyns in Park City, Utah, yet at the time I was the only one serving a population of nearly 35,000! Furthermore, I did not do obstetrics—only gynecology.

When I called the committee chairman, he explained that they assumed I was going to retire and would no longer see patients near one of "their" hospitals. I told him that just the opposite was the case. I would be seeing lots of patients in a place that was very close to several of "his" hospitals. Within two weeks, I was told that this HMO could not verify what I had said and so the termination held. Yet as far as I know, no one at the office where I was seeing patients received a call from this HMO. In the last letter I received from the HMO director, he acknowledged that I had unique skills that set me apart from other doctors and for this reason, I was allowed to see some of "their" patients on referral from other physicians, but only if the referring physician obtained permission in advance from them. Guess how many times that occurred? Zero. Subsequently, when I called to confirm this arrangement, I was told that they knew of no such agreement. This is HMO medicine at its finest.

## It Just Doesn't Add Up

According to the *New England Journal of Medicine,* the United States government currently spends nearly $4,000 per person/per year for health care—a figure that is substantially higher than other countries. In fact, annual health care spending in the United States may be close to $3 trillion in less than ten years. We have the dubious distinction of having the most costly and one of the most inefficient health care systems in the world. (What a distinction.)

Japan outshines the United States in virtually *every health category,* including available MRI (magnetic resonance imaging) units and computed tomography scanners, yet their health care costs are a fraction of ours. Moreover, drugs cost about 60 percent less in Europe than they do here, and European firms spend more of their revenues on research and development than their American counterparts. American drug firms would rather spend money on marketing schemes. And if research trials are conducted, one has to ask whose agenda was furthered by the study.

## The Truth about Clinical Research

Thomas Bodenheimer, author of the *New England Journal of*

*Medicine* article "Uneasy Alliance—Clinical Investigators and the Pharmaceutical Industry," points out that most clinical studies which bring new drugs from bench to bedside are financed by pharmaceutical companies. In fact, seventy percent of the money provided for clinical drug trials in the United States comes from the pharmaceutical industry rather than from the National Institutes of Health (NIH). With physicians adding new pharmacologic weapons to their therapeutic armamentarium every day, Bodenheimer asks this million-dollar question: "Can practicing physicians trust the information they receive about the medications they are prescribing?"

The barrage of new drug data doctors must sort through boggles the mind. Pharmaceutical sales representatives continually bombard physicians with scores of new drugs and their corresponding literature. Doctors are expected to immediately assimilate these drugs into their treatment armory and dispense them as soon as possible. How can any physician stay updated on the risks and contraindications of every drug? Consequently, doctors assume that if a drug has a decent track record, they can dole it out without reservations.

A nurse who used to work for me is now a pharmaceutical sales rep. She tells me that "pharm reps" have assumed the responsibility for educating physicians on the merits of new drugs, and that doctors usually trust that their information is accurate. Who are we fooling here? Since when did sales reps become qualified to teach doctors the benefits and dangers of drugs? Reps are there to sell, not educate! During one of these "orientations," my former nurse heard another rep proclaim to a doctor that a drug for menopause didn't need to address vaginal atrophy because the condition didn't exist. Having been a gynecologic nurse for several years, she challenged his claim and informed him that atrophy was indeed a legitimate disorder that she had seen for herself. If this is a sampling of the type of misinformation exchanged between reps and doctors, we're in big trouble!

Not unexpectedly, drug reps stopped calling me when I began preaching prevention and the use of nonprescription medication. I learned that they didn't like reversing roles and having me "educate" them.

# Doctors, Drugs and Indoctrination

Voltaire put it this way, "Doctors are men who prescribe medicines of which they know little, to cure diseases of which they know less, in human beings of whom they know nothing." Perhaps this characterization is a bit harsh, but it sheds much needed light on practices within the profession that need to be exposed. For example, pharmaceutical companies routinely recruit young interns and begin their indoctrination early. A recent report in *Lancet* points out that drug companies exert a considerable influence on students in medical school. The effect is subtle at first—a logo on a pen, a trade name on a medical bag, then perhaps an all-expense paid trip to a symposium in an exotic city, etc. etc. In fact, the *Journal of the American Medical Association* reports that pharmaceutical companies spend more than $11 billion each year to promote and market drugs—an estimated $8,000 to $13,000 per physician/per year. The money comes in the form of meals, lodging, entertainment, books and even medical supplies.

You better believe this has an impact on what doctors choose to prescribe and how often they scribble it on their prescription forms! A 2000 study on the subject concluded that doctors' decisions regarding what to prescribe are indeed influenced by the gifts and perks they accept from pharmaceutical companies.

In fact, according to a February 2003 Associated Press report, New York Attorney General Eliot Spitzer has given notice of its intent to file suit against three major pharmaceutical companies who he says are giving illegal incentives to doctors and pharma-

cists to favor their products. These "under the counter" entice-
ments are supposedly driving up prescriptions costs and setting
back New Yorkers between $50 and $100 million annually,
according to Spitzer. Although the companies deny any wrong
doing, Texas and California have already taken similar legislative
measures. How can you draw the line on what is ethically per-
missible in my profession when the boundaries keep shifting?

# Drugs Can Kill

According to the American Medical Association's own data,
scores of Americans die every year from drugs they were
instructed to take by their doctors. At a recent Congressional
hearing on the safety of dietary supplements, Dan Burton,
Republican representative and advocate for alternative therapies,
made it known that over one hundred thousand people died in
one year from prescription drugs as opposed to forty-two thousand in automobile accidents and sixteen deaths from the use of
dietary supplements. Still, you can bet your bottom dollar that if
someone gets a hangnail from using a dietary supplement, it
makes the six o'clock news. Make no mistake, the pharmaceutical lobby continues to drive potential legislation that will negatively affect the status of dietary supplements.

One example of this bias is the controversy currently swirling
around the herb ephedra, also known as ma huang. Ephedra is
the main ingredient used in a number of popular weight-loss
products. According to the FDA, ephedra has been implicated in
a number of adverse effects ranging from disabilities to death,
but what is the real truth here? Have people really died as a direct
result of taking ephedra? While no one disputes that ephedra-
containing products should be used judiciously, recent deaths or
side effects associated with ephedra may have well been caused
by some other health condition or interaction. According to

some figures, *more than 3 billion doses* of ephedra were consumed in 1999, putting the incidence of adverse events at *less than one-thousandth of one percent.* Compare that to known deaths and serious side effects associated with over-the-counter or prescription drugs.

Ephedra products generally contain an extract comprising 6–8 percent alkaloids (ephedrine and pseudoephedrine) that are considered stimulants, and any stimulatory compound should be used with caution. Keep in mind that scores of cold and asthma remedies that line grocery store and pharmacy shelves contain synthetically produced versions of the same alkaloids found in ephedra. Ephedrine constricts blood vessels and speeds the heart rate. Pseudoephedrine dilates bronchiole tubes and eases nasal congestion. These products are readily available and rarely come under any public scrutiny, (in spite of the fact that some of them are routinely purchased to produce illegal methamphetamine drugs).

Any product containing these compounds (herbal or not) can interact with other medications and should not be abused or taken in large doses. While this has been known for years, I don't see the FDA yanking cold tablets and cough syrups containing ephedrine or pseudoephedrine off store shelves. The potential health hazards of product side effects, interactions and inconsistent potency or contamination are a problem for many herbs and medicines across the board. My gripe is that while the dangers of ephedra make the news headlines, nobody seems to blink an eye that thousands of people die from adverse effects of prescription drugs. The annual cost of prescription drug-related injury and deaths (doctor and ER visits, as well as additional prescriptions and long-term care) in the United States is over $76 billion. It reminds me of an old saying by Moliere uttered in the 1600s, "Nearly all men die of their medicines, not of their diseases."

Many women agree to take powerful prescription drugs without knowing all of the facts. For instance, if a gynecologist wants to put a woman on a potent drug like Lupron for endometriosis, she needs to fully understand how that drug will impact her body before taking it. Mixing drugs can also be dangerous. If a woman is taking a high blood pressure medication, Prozac, birth control pills and a sleep aid, she could find herself experiencing a number of side effects that her physician neglected to mention (or was unaware of).

Moreover, the ill effects of many drugs may not be discovered for years. At least one in five new drugs has serious side effects that don't show up until well after receiving FDA approval, according to an April 2002 issue of *JAMA*. Consider this— approximately 20 percent of the new drugs researchers studied had to be given serious side effect warnings or were taken off the market.

The DES tragedy is the perfect example of the kind of devastating damage a seemingly benign drug can do. Potentially serious side effects from drugs can slip through the cracks for years. The links between aspirin and Reye's syndrome, NSAIDs and stomach damage, and Phen-fen and heart valve destruction took years to surface. Consider the following examples:

- Seldane, the most popular allergy medication worldwide during the last decade, stayed on the market for almost ten years after the drug was found to be dangerous to the heart. It was removed from the market by the FDA in 1997.

- Propulsid, prescribed for heartburn, stayed on the market for seven years despite scores of reported heart arrhythmias and several deaths before it was finally withdrawn.

- The makers of Baycol (cerivastatin), a popular cholesterol-lowering drug used by about 700,000 Americans, pulled their product off the market in 2001 due to numerous deaths and muscle paralysis linked to its use. Also, some doctors have

## Drug Costs: Gouging the Consumer

□ ▪ ▪ ▪

A recent report by investigative reporter Steve Wilson in Michigan sheds new light on how some pharmacies cash in on the generic drug market. He discovered that the cost of generic drugs (which are supposed to save you money) can greatly vary, depending on where you do your shopping. "We went to store after store after store where a prescription for a generic that costs the pharmacy only about $2 is being sold to many of you for as much as $100, despite their denials."

He uses generic Prozac as an example. A thirty-day supply of the generic version of Prozac is a prescription that costs drugstores only $2.16 or less. Keep in mind that a month's supply of the name-brand Prozac sells for about $100. Consequently, some drugstores sell the generic for $92.24 and still have the nerve to tell the consumer that they're "saving a few bucks." Talk about unethical. According to Wilson, "The truth is no matter where we went, from the big chain drug stores to the independent, to the pharmacies at Krogers and Farmer Jacks, even to the so-called discounters like Meijer and Wal-Mart and Kmart, too, we found to one degree or another, much if not most of the potential savings on generics are going into the till at the pharmacy." The only exception was the pharmacy at Costco where Wilson found that, "On each and every one of the drugs we checked, it was the pharmacy at Costco that was not only cheaper, but dramatically far and away cheaper than everyone across the Metro area. While that other pharmacy is charging $92 for generic Prozac, Costco is selling it for $9. When the chain stores sell generic Pepcid for close to $100, Costco is dispensing it for only about $12." This kind of discrepancy in generic drug pricing is criminal and should be regulated. For the person on a fixed income, the difference in dollars is enormous.

known that other cholesterol-lowering drugs can cause serious muscle inflammation in some patients but failed to warn them.

• Rezulin, a medication used for diabetes, was found to have potentially lethal side effects and was taken off the market in Great Britain in 1997, but it was still available for purchase in the U.S. until 2000, after it was associated with sixty-three confirmed deaths.

I'm not saying that all drugs are damaging. I am saying that doctors, pharmaceutical companies and the FDA need more judicious guidelines governing how drugs are dispensed. After all, the consequences of the careless or casual dispensing of drugs are patient harm and time spent in court—an expensive exercise that raises the cost of medicine for everyone.

## Maude's Mixed Bag of Medicines

Maude, a sixty-two-year-old woman who was short for her weight and did not exercise, came to seem me recently for pelvic pain, diarrhea, epigastric distress and overall weakness. The list of prescriptions she was taking could have filled an eight by eleven inch sheet of paper. She was taking pills for high cholesterol, acid reflux (at twice the recommended dosage), high blood pressure (which she didn't even have), depression, and osteoporosis (which she also did not have), as well as taking HRT, sleeping pills and an assortment of vitamins and other remedies.

When I asked her how much money the drugs cost her, she said that her co-pay was fifty dollars a month with the actual cost being eight hundred dollars each month. After reviewing the side effects of these medications, I discovered that most of her problems were caused by the drugs she was taking! After decreasing the dosages of many of her medications (or halting them altogether) and putting her on my program (regular exercise, a better diet and a few supplements), many of her symptoms have disappeared—without compromising her health.

# Drugs, Natural Products and Insurance Coverage

Pharmaceutical drugs cost about 60 percent less in Europe than they do here. American prescription medicine costs give new meaning to the notion of "sticker shock." But there is something even more insidious going on here than simply gouging consumers. Most insurance plans have drug co-pays, right? The co-pay system may seem like a good thing, but what people don't understand is that while they think the prescription is only costing them a few dollars, they have no idea what the drug actually costs the entire system. And here's the kicker—while your insurance company covers the cost of an expensive statin drug to control your cholesterol, it won't cover a much less expensive but equally effective red yeast rice supplement. So, if you're strapped for money, you'll actually end up paying less out of your own pocket for the prescription drug. This is ludicrous.

Although some HMOs are beginning to see the light and now offer discounts for some unconventional treatments and other preventive measures, many others refuse to acknowledge the value of sound nutritional practices in preventing the biggest (and most expensive) killers of our time—heart attacks, cancer, stroke and Alzheimer's disease.

How many doctors does it take to screw in a light bulb? It depends on whether the light bulb has health insurance! In all seriousness, today's medical practices are directly linked to their coverage schedule. These means that insurance companies would rather pay for outrageously priced drugs with major side effects than for safe, less-expensive, nonpharmaceutical medicines. The good news is that some insurance companies are beginning to cover the cost of complementary treatments backed by credible data. To be fair to insurance companies, most natural products or dietary supplements lack standardized quality controls, making it very difficult to distinguish real medicine from snake oil (which is why dealing with reputable companies and professionals is so important). Yes, we need to be concerned about proper standardization, unfounded claims, side effects, and related issues, but we must also scrutinize pharmaceuticals in the same way.

Chapter 3

□ ▨ ▪ ▪

# Women and Bias: Getting the Short End of the Stick

*"I never doubted that equal rights was the right direction.
Most reforms, most problems, are complicated. But to me there
is nothing complicated about ordinary equality.*
*Alice Paul*

**If you're an** American woman, you belong to a group of people who aren't getting their fair share of medical care. Simply stated, doctors have not been adequately educated on female physiology—consequently many of them misunderstand or worse yet, minimize hormone-driven maladies. Whether physicians admit it or not, an undercurrent of skepticism and dismissal toward women has permeated the medical establishment. I'll never forget what one of my patients shared with me, "Dr. Townsend, my former doctor never took my PMS symptoms seriously and yet when my husband goes in for a hangnail, he gets his undivided attention." Let me interject here that medical students simply aren't educated regarding the changing hormonal landscape of women and how it impacts every aspect of their health. A good gynecologist recognizes that women face unique biological challenges and that each woman is different. The "one size fits all" approach to HRT is a good example of what happens when research methodologies are inherently flawed and doctors make blanket assumptions about menopause.

Women have lost the most under today's health care system, particularly in the area of cancer care. I can say without hesitation that the medical establishment fails to diagnose too many cancers. Consequently, in some states, malpractice rates have increased dramatically due to these oversights. Ironically, most of these errors didn't occur because of doctor incompetence, but rather because a proper evaluation of the condition wasn't made for one reason or another. In other words, time and money.

One of the major roles of a gynecologist is to provide women with direction and sound advice. Unfortunately, our current system discourages the role of doctor as advisor. HMO-imposed time constraints are especially damaging to women who, according to the Henry J. Kaiser Foundation in Washington, D.C., are more likely to need ongoing medical treatment than men. In fact, a recent phone survey from the Foundation found that 22 percent of women were dissatisfied with the quality of health care they were currently receiving, and one in seven women ranked their health insurance plan and the quality of physicians on their plan as very poor. Any other industry with ratings this low would eventually go down the drain.

## Gender Bias: The Shocking Facts

According to the Commonwealth Fund's September 2000 *Issue Brief* on women's health, only one-quarter of women over sixty-five and half of younger women see an ob/gyn, despite the fact that women with a gynecologist are more likely to receive thorough preventative care.

Too many health plans require a woman to see her already overworked primary care physician before she can go to a gynecologist or other specialist. This is lunacy. Not only is it a waste of time, it can be dangerous as well. Jumping through HMO hoops takes time—precious time—during which undetected tumors can grow and metastasize. In addition, a general practitioner can misdiagnose or completely miss a serious condition. For example, a recent study in the *Journal of the American College of Chest Physicians* found that primary care physicians were more likely to misdiagnose women with chronic obstructive lung disease. Physicians correctly diagnosed the disease (which is the fourth leading cause of death in the U.S.) in men 64 percent of the time, but only 49 percent of the time in women, although women are more susceptible to it. Women with the disease were often told they had asthma.

Women may also be shortchanged when it comes to reducing their risk of heart disease (the number-one killer of women), according to a study in the *Archives of Internal Medicine*. The nationwide study, which followed American men and women from 1994 to 1997, was designed to look at the effects of a blood pressure medication on cholesterol. Researchers discovered that doctors undertreat women with high cholesterol. In other words, more men than women are given cholesterol-lowering medication.

A 1991 study in the *New England Journal of Medicine* further illustrates the gender bias that exists in treating heart disease. In 1999, almost 50 percent of women who had a heart attack died within a year, as opposed to only 27 percent of men. Why? Doctors spot cardiovascular red flags sooner in men and treat them more aggressively. This is a shameful statistic. Even worse is this: between the ages of forty and sixty-five, close to five hundred thousand women die each year from heart-related disorders.

Even if a woman is fortunate enough to find a good doctor, she may still be sabotaged by her insurance provider. HMOs are notorious for notifying a patient without warning that they must switch to another physician. When a woman's insurance plan changes, she may need to change both her primary care physician and gynecologist. Because the personal investment women

## Claim: Denied

☐ ■ ■ ■

What is the major goal of an HMO? Sometimes I feel that it's to deny as many claims as possible. And women are denied medical care more often than men are. According to researchers out of the University of Cleveland, the University of Michigan and the Urban Institute in Washington, D.C., the average man has a 25 to 30 percent better chance of getting a kidney transplant than the average woman. Yet men make up just slightly more than half of those suffering from end-stage renal disease. Women on kidney transplant waiting lists in 1999 waited nearly three years longer than men for a transplant. They also waited more than two months longer for hearts and receive a mere 27 percent of heart transplants, although heart disease is the number-one killer in both men and women.

A number of studies have also shown that male-specific medical procedures are reimbursed at higher rates than female-specific ones. One study examined the ten most common illnesses eligible for reimbursement. It found that three of four illnesses with the highest out-of-pocket expense were more common in women, and four out of five illnesses with the lowest out-of-pocket cost were most common in men. A follow-up study found that male-specific procedures were reimbursed up to 44 percent higher than comparable female-specific procedures (found to be similar in level of difficulty and time investment). For instance, a penile biopsy was reimbursed 36 percent higher than a biopsy of the vulva. And a procedure that involves removing part of the prostate was valued 164 percent higher than endometrial ablation.

Here's another example of gender inequity. In the last few years, Viagra has taken the country by storm. You can bet that when it comes to the treatment of male impotence, most insurance companies will cover its cost. By contrast, coverage for mammograms, birth control pills, diaphragms, treatments for osteoporosis, and so on, are often restricted or completely rejected. Although gender gaps have narrowed as a result of raised awareness, inequalities still exist—including limits to health care for the elderly, which adversely affects more women than men because women live longer.

make in their doctors is sizeable, when the fit between a woman and her doctor is good (like a comfortable shoe), it's often traumatic to make a change. In addition, if she switches insurance providers, she may also experience gaps in coverage. According to 1998 statistics, more than one in four women were uninsured at some time during the year, and half of uninsured women had no coverage for over a year. I don't know about you, but I get angry when I read statistics like this.

## The Devaluing of Women

I'm angry that woman have been subjected to substandard medical care for decades. Until 1992, with the creation of the Women's Health Initiative, women were completely excluded from numerous major clinical trials. (Despite the fact that most drug studies show gender differences due to changing hormone levels in women.) Clearly, the bulk of research has been skewed toward diseases that afflict men. To add insult to injury, since many textbooks only describe clinical symptoms of diseases as they occur in men, women with major health problems may not be properly diagnosed. For instance, the CDC definition for AIDS did not include gynecological symptoms like cervical cancer until 1993. As a result, doctors failed to diagnose the disease early on in many women, and HIV-positive women without classical male symptoms were often denied services and insurance coverage, according to the Society for the Advancement of Women's Health Research.

Even more disturbing is information from the Council on Graduate Medical Education, which reported in 1995 that physicians were not prepared to competently provide care for women. In fact, the report called for major changes in the scope and content of med school classes on women's health. It also called for more gender-specific research and the cultivation of more women in leadership positions in academic medicine. What a wake-up call!

Simply stated, women's health issues are largely different than men's. Although they may live longer, women suffer from more conditions than men (such as depression, osteoporosis, carpal tunnel, and migraines). The hormonal havoc caused by the estrogen/progesterone seesaw cannot be minimized. It must be treated by doctors who understand the wide health implications it has for women. Our overall failure to do so is reprehensible.

The "good ol' boy" approach to medicine has neglected to address women's health issues. Many victimized women accept the status quo or worse yet, stop going to the doctor altogether. For this reason, women have the most to gain from medical reform. Doctors won't see the light until they feel the heat. So women, muster your forces! Ask questions, and raise your expectations! If you don't speak up, who will?

Finally, we need to recruit more women into the medical profession. Someone once told me that a male gynecologist is like an auto mechanic that never owned a car! Although more women are entering the field as doctors, currently only 20 to 25 percent of the American College of Obstetricians and Gynecologists are women. So, talk to your doctor and write letters to the American Medical Association, your HMOs and to your local newspapers. You can prompt reform only if you take action. It is the right of every woman to be treated by caring, sensitive and compassionate doctors who listen with open minds and do their homework when it comes to finding the best treatments, conventional or alternative.

## The HMO Runaround for Susan

Less than a year after my first snag with an insurance provider, I had a similar experience with another well-known HMO. Susan, another patient of mine, needed surgical repair for a prolapse, and I explained to her that I would only do the surgery at a hospital that was not approved by her HMO. I called the local medical director of Susan's HMO and explained the new procedure I felt would best remedy her problem. Although he seemed receptive to my proposal, a week later he called to tell me that she did not need the operation. If she opted to have it anyway, I would have to do it at one of their hospitals. He recommended that I do a different procedure— one that had a 30 percent chance of failing.

After the phone call, I met with Susan and her husband and told them that I would not perform the surgery suggested by their HMO, nor would I return to a hospital where I had experienced so many problems. Susan decided to petition her husband's employer so I would be allowed to do the best procedure for her problem at the hospital of my choice, and eventually we got the go-ahead. The surgery was successful. Four years later, Susan remains healthy and problem-free.

Two weeks following her surgery, however, I received a phone call from the local medical director of her HMO informing me that I was being dropped from their panel without any explanation. I later discovered that an HMO can drop any physician without cause. This would not be the last HMO to drop me from their rolls for putting patients first.

## Breast Cancer, Inc.: The Corporate Cash-In

☐ ▨ ▧ ▧

It's easy to see how pharmaceutical companies and HMOs are manipulating health care for profit, but companies not directly linked to health care are also cashing in on current health concerns. In fact, more and more of them have developed marketing plans that link their corporate identities to "hot" health issues. While many businesses generate money for research, just as many exploit disease for profit. Because the threat of breast cancer pushes everyone's buttons, companies that supply food, appliances, clothing and cosmetics are all jumping on the bandwagon and increasing their sales by claiming that proceeds go toward "finding a cure." Don't get me wrong. Some of this money may actually find its way to the coffers of breast cancer research, but the truth is no one really knows how much actually gets there.

One thing is clear—we haven't found a cure for breast cancer. In fact, more women are getting breast cancer each year in spite of the billions spent on diagnosis, treatment and research. Unfortunately, breast cancer's "pretty in pink" makeover has done little to change its grim reality. Granted, corporate America has every right to cash in on the emotion that breast cancer creates, but it doesn't have the right to imply that its motives are completely altruistic. They're not. Turf struggles over breast cancer campaigns can be just as nasty as marketing plans not linked to a "worthy" cause. Madison avenue knows that the little pink ribbon inspires a very lucrative brand of loyalty from consumers.

Using our free enterprise system to fund cancer research is fine and dandy, but it should be seen for what it is. While companies push their products under the banner of pink, money is often drained away from heart disease and lung cancer research, which each kill more women every year than breast cancer. Equally important is the fact that little money goes into breast cancer prevention—one of the best ways to lower its incidence. Let me reiterate—I'm not saying that corporations or individuals for that matter shouldn't give charitable donations to cancer research. What I am saying is that before we open our wallets, we need to know how much of our money actually gets to the cause and how much goes to company profit.

## We Need Real Reform

Lawsuits against the medical industry are becoming commonplace, and the call for reform is intensifying. Case in point—in one high-profile lawsuit against an HMO in 1996, a California widow was awarded a record $116 million in punitive damages after her husband died as a result of his HMO denying him coverage for a new cancer treatment. This industry's violations against its users are so blatantly egregious that the United States Congress was compelled to construct a "bill of rights" to protect you and me from abuse.

We can talk about managed health care accountability until we're blue in the face, but it doesn't change the facts. HMOs by their very nature and mission statements are dictatorial and self-serving businesses spawned by misguided governmental intervention. Congress passed the HMO Act in 1973 and nothing has been right since. For example, your doctor must be familiar with over one hundred thousand pages of Medicare red tape, where even the tiniest oversight can result in fines and prison time. Freedom from this kind of choke hold would free up the medical system to correct itself. The last thing we need is more government intervention. What we need is more doctor-patient time, house calls, better insurance coverage and reasonable medical costs. When a system is this badly broken, it doesn't need repair—it needs to be scrapped altogether. And women can help stimulate change. How? As someone once said, "I know you don't make the laws, but I also know that you are the wives and mothers, the sisters and daughters of those who do."

## The Managed Care Alternative

Other managed care programs, like preferred provider organizations (PPOs), are becoming more popular since they give the patient more freedom of choice. Large PPOs list hundreds of physicians that patients can choose from. However, most PPOs and other managed care programs are still for-profit, and a substantial amount of money is spent on administrative costs rather than health care.

Obviously there is no ideal health insurance plan, but letting the marketplace dictate health care is a terrible idea and does not work. Likewise, government involvement bogs down health care in bureaucracy and makes it susceptible to legislative agendas (where the primary concern is re-election). So what is my solution? I don't know how to fix "the system," but I do know that when we are healthy, we aren't subject to the whims of our drug companies, HMOs, doctors, or even our insurance providers. The best way for you to take charge of your health destiny is to adopt a healthy lifestyle. Preventing disease keeps the cost of health care down for everyone.

□ ■ ■ ■

# Chapter 4

# Prevention: The Best Medicine

Modern medicine is a negation of health. It isn't organized
to serve human health, but only itself, as an institution.
It makes more people sick than it heals.
*– Ivan Illich (medical historian)*

**In 1994, I** found myself sitting in a run-of-the mill hotel conference room watching a short, nondescript "doctor" take the podi-
um (in those days anyone who called themselves a doctor without a medical degree was considered a quack). He was a "naturopath," and to make things worse, I found him annoyingly effu-
sive. Naturally, I assumed that he was terribly uneducated and
misguided, but I was nevertheless willing to listen because I
wanted to find out all I could to keep my cancer at bay. The simple fact was that if the cancer did return, it would probably kill
me. So, I was ready to consider all forms of prevention.

As the doctor began talking about nutrition, I began to lose
focus. That is until he dropped this bombshell, "There are more
bacteria in your gut than cells in your body." He now had my
undivided attention. Why? Because he knew something I didn't,
and that was unacceptable to me.

This was the first of many encounters in which I discussed the value of natural therapies with this man. It became obvious that he knew more about cellular biochemistry than I did, and for this reason, he understood how natural compounds impact chemical reactions in the human body. "You see, Duane," he said, "You can't just add toxic chemicals to the body and expect it to get well—you must prompt the body to sharpen its own biochemical reactions and you do that with substances it will recognize." While this guy wasn't a trained medical doctor, he sure knew his stuff. So much so that a major cancer treatment center asked him to design an herbal formula that would boost the immune system of cancer patients and enhance their response to chemotherapy and radiation. I quickly realized that this man's knowledge could help me prevent my own cancer from returning. And so I picked his brain. "What foods best fight cancer?" "Give me your ten best anticancer supplements." "How can I maximize my own internal defense mechanisms?" and so forth. There was no turning back now. I was on my way to embracing alternative medicine, and I would be the guinea pig.

My curiosity would lead me into the remarkable world of natural compounds like genistein, a compound found in soybeans, red clover and kudzu that possesses estrogen-like properties. After reviewing the hundreds of studies on genistein, I told my wife that it would one day assume a prominent place in our health world. As of this writing, that prediction continues to become a reality. In view of new concerns raised about the dangers of hormone replacement therapy, the role of natural alternatives—like genistein—for women is now considered a crucial one.

Believe me, I was very familiar with the shortcomings of conventional care, especially in the areas of cancer and women's health. So I began exploring other unconventional ways of fighting disease. I researched anything and everything—mind-body theories, biofeedback, macrobiotic diets, Chinese herbal medicine, apple cider vinegar, colon cleansing—you name it, I read about it. My appetite for new and better healthy therapies was growing daily. Of course, I was not automatically impressed by everything I read (in fact, much of it was garbage). I spent countless frustrating hours in university libraries, on the phone, and reviewing medical journals. One thing was clear—the conventional medical world had little to offer in the way of disease prevention. But slowly I began to see that good health is a complex mix of many different factors, many of which were not taught to me in med school. It was painfully apparent that I had a lot to learn.

# The Practice of Principled Medicine

I like the old saying, "If you can't stand the heat get out of the kitchen," because my kitchen has always been hot. You better believe that suggesting complementary treatments to my patients has rattled a few cages. (I can't tell you how many of my fellow doctors think I've lost it.) The remarkable trend toward unconventional medicine has prompted the merger of traditional medicine with complementary therapies—hence a new term has emerged called "integrative medicine," which means using the best of all worlds to promote health and fight disease.

Call this new emerging mode of health care whatever you want—integrative, natural, complementary—that's not important. What's important is that we acknowledge that patients are not happy with the status quo. They want more than drugs or surgery options. And what I want is the best way to help the women who trust me. While many physicians are too hardheaded to consider alternatives to modern medical practices, the tried and true principles of lasting health are nothing new. For centuries they have been based on the following:

• the healing power of the body
• doing no harm to the patient

• identifying and treating the cause of disease, not just its symptoms
• promoting the role of health practitioner as teacher and healer
• preventing disease

Eleven years ago, I was on an airplane, nervously awaiting a phone call. For years, my wife had been bugging me to check out an odd-looking mole on my shoulder, telling me it could be cancer. I put her off, though deep down I was afraid that it might really be that bad. Finally, I relented and had the mole removed and sent in for analysis. And now I was leaving town, feeling certain the next phone call I took could change my life.

"Duane, I hate to tell you this, but it is cancer," the pathologist told me. Though it's exactly what I expected, I was nevertheless stunned. Shock soon turned to terror. The type of cancer he was describing was a pernicious, even deadly form—malignant melanoma. I knew I was in for the fight of my life.

Immediately, I had to consider my options, fearful that the available treatments would not be enough to prevent a recurrence. It was during this time and the next several years that I became convinced of one thing: the best way that I could have beat my cancer—or any other disease, for that matter—would have been to prevent it in the first place. That's right. These are truly words to live by: *preventing disease is the best way to treat disease.*

Of course, there are no guarantees that we can absolutely prevent any disease, especially cancer. But there are bookshelves of data showing that we can drastically cut our risks for disease with simple preventive measures—things like eating a well-rounded diet, getting adequate sleep, exercising a couple times a week, not smoking or drinking alcohol, managing stress, minimizing the toxins in our environment, taking nutritional supplements, having a regular (and thorough) physical exam, and engaging in meaningful relationships with family and friends.

For some of us, that may require a monumental change of lifestyle. But it's worth it. If you choose to ignore your health, rest assured it will eventually catch up with you in the form of diabetes, arthritis, osteoporosis, heart disease, cancer and a myriad of other conditions. In fact, so many Americans are affected by these illnesses that they have become expected, almost normal, consequences of aging. In truth, they are most often the consequence of poor lifestyle choices.

As a physician, my top priority is this—to stop disease before it even starts. Whether you call it "natural," "integrative," "conventional" or "unconventional," if it has merit, I'm interested. I really don't care what it's called. I simply want what works best and is safest for my patients.

## Disease Prevention = Bad Business

We are a sick nation. "What are you talking about?" you're probably asking. Some argue that we are living longer than ever. This is true. But what is also true is that our later years are spent in misery from a number of "natural" ailments, taking handfuls of drugs three times a day, recovering from quadruple bypass surgery or chemotherapy, and having the doctor tell us repeatedly that "Sorry, there really isn't any more that we can do." Simply put, we aren't living healthier, we're only prolonging our poor health.

America currently spends almost $4,000 per person, per year on health care. Japan spends less than $2,000, and the average Japanese person lives five years longer than we do. Cubans live almost as long as Americans, yet their government spends only $500 per person annually on health care. Is it just me, or is there a problem here? Health care spending in the U.S. is projected to top $2.8 trillion by 2011, controlling an even larger chunk of the nation's gross domestic product (GDP) than previously forecast. If these projections are true, annual health care spending will rise to $9,216 per person, per year—twice the amount spent per capita in 2000. Some experts put it this way: health costs will one day exceed our gross domestic product. *Wow.*

This begs the question—are we getting our money's worth? Trillions of dollars will be spent on diagnostic procedures, disease treatment and prescription drugs, yet we are becoming more and more sick—lifestyle diseases like diabetes, heart disease and extreme obesity (especially among children) are rapidly rising. We have also seen the emergence of various "mystery" diseases like chronic fatigue syndrome, fibromyalgia and vulvodynia, a condition that affects more than a million women. Most of our money goes to treat diseases after the fact. Very few dollars fund prevention.

Naturally, we all must share some of the blame. Too many of us refuse to incorporate preventive health measures into our lifestyle. Instead we continue to rely on the "magic pill" mentality, wanting only drugs that mask our symptoms and temporarily make us feel better. As Adele Davis, a pioneer in using diet to promote wellness, said in 1954, "Thousands upon thousands of persons have studied disease. Almost no one has studied health."

## No Profits in Prevention

If medicine were living up to its stewardship to safeguard health, it would be, as James Bryce said, "the only profession that labors incessantly to destroy the reason for its own existence." But that isn't the case, especially in this country. As I mentioned earlier, Japanese people spend considerably less on health care than we do, yet they live healthier and longer lives. Why the difference? It's simple—the Japanese eat better and exercise more regularly. It's called prevention, that little-known notion that has never caught on here. And why should it? Consider this quote from the British Cancer Control Society about what influences cancer care: "Economics and politics simply intertwine in shaping conventional medicine's approach to cancer." It doesn't take a rocket scientist to figure out a major conflict of interest exists within various areas of the medical establishment, especially the pharmaceutical industry. If they were to push the idea of preventing disease with a healthy lifestyle, they would lose money (and I mean lots of money) because their drugs and other services would not be prescribed. (If you're skeptical about all this, read the Chapter 2, which discusses HMOs and the pharmaceutical industry.) Simply put, treating disease—not preventing it—makes these people a lot of money.

## Scientific Proof that Prevention Is Better

The truth is that there are mountains of data showing that preventive measures—modifying one's diet, increasing physical activity, reducing stress levels, taking nutritional supplements and the like—can have a tremendous benefit on your health. For instance, dozens of studies detail how increasing your intake of B vitamins lowers your risk of heart disease. Many more detail how moderate exercise can significantly cut the incidence of type II diabetes. And expert after expert agrees that reducing stress levels can decreases your chances of stroke. Despite this, the focus of research and education funds is largely placed on developing and promoting after-the-fact treatments—that is, drugs and surgery.

Here's a great example of what I'm talking about. I'm sure you've seen news reports lately of the huge number of people—including kids—that are currently diagnosed with type II diabetes. Nearly 10 percent of Americans now have the disease, which is nothing less than a major epidemic (and those numbers continue to rise). Type II diabetes occurs when cells become unable to respond properly to insulin (the chemical that regulates blood sugar levels). No matter what some doctors may say, the best way to avoid the disease is to minimize risk factors such as obesity. Not surprisingly, according to the *New England Journal of Medicine,* a healthy lifestyle is actually a more effective treatment for type II diabetes than drug therapy. The February 2002 issue features a study where the use of glucophage—a common diabetes drug used to control blood-sugar levels—was compared to exercise and dietary changes. Researchers concluded that the test subjects who improved their lifestyles—principally in the areas of nutrition and physical activity—had a 58 percent lower risk of developing type II diabetes than people in the placebo group. Those given glucophage cut their diabetes risk by only 31 percent. Sure, you could say it's difficult to eat better, exercise a little, and turn off the tube. But it's worth the effort—you'll be healthier and happier.

## The Immune Wars

Of course, diabetes isn't the only disease where prevention plays a major role. Cancer organizations spend millions on advertising for early detection (which is important), but virtually nothing on prevention research or education. We know how we should eat to prevent cancer, so why aren't we getting the word out? We know that our immune systems play a crucial role in preventing cancer (and a bunch of other diseases), but physicians spend very little time teaching their patients how to boost their immunity.

Case in point. There are a number of "natural" compounds—including astragalus, vitamins C and A, zinc, beta glucan, olive leaf extract, and echinacea—that have scores of studies backing their ability to improve immune function. One supplement in particular—called transfer factor—is supported by mountains of research data. This promising compound can actually add defense information to our immune "data banks," which ultimately enhances the ability of our immune systems to fight cancerous cells, pathogens, and other dangerous toxins.

I have reviewed the literature on transfer factor and use it with hundreds of my patients. I've seen first-hand the impressive results that transfer factor produces. In light of this, I have to ask myself, "Why isn't transfer factor used by medical doctors?" Granted, many doctors have never heard of it. But even those who have heard of it display the usual mix of bias, ignorance and skepticism of unconventional therapies. I've explained the health benefits of transfer factor to dozens of doctors, yet all I get is a polite smile and casual dismissal punctuated with words like "unproven," "that's interesting," or even "harmful." And remember folks—these are the same doctors that write out hundreds of prescriptions every year for cold and flu drugs that may provide some relief from annoying symptoms, but often prolong the infection and do nothing to prevent it from occurring again next month.

## A Total Transformation

When Nancy came to see me, she was suffering from some pretty horrible symptoms—heavy periods, PMS, headaches, breast tenderness and other signs typical of an estrogen overload. She had gone to several doctors and tried everything they recommended. Although she came in expecting just a brief exam and perhaps a few suggestions for supplements, I gave her my diet "lecture" and we developed a personalized exercise plan as well.

Nancy did just as I advised—she changed her diet, began exercising and took the "dynamic duo" of genistein and natural progesterone. The results were dramatic. She had lost considerable weight and her symptoms essentially vanished. In addition, her sex drive improved, and her fibrocystic breast disease disappeared. Yes, I said disappeared. Remember that she accomplished all of this without the use of drugs or surgery. Just another case where preventive/

unconventional measures won out over drugs, surgery, or whatever else the establishment had to offer.

## Proof Pros and Cons

If you cared to count, my name appears on a number of published studies and articles. I'm painfully aware of research methodologies, with all of their pros and cons. I learned early in my career that gathering data to support a premise is extremely important. So if you want to talk to me about a supplemental treatment, show me the data! Convince me with facts and I'll listen, but I won't hesitate to shoot down faulty claims or assumptions about any remedy.

On the other hand, I've also learned to take any scientific "evidence" used to prove a claim with a grain of salt—whether for or against nontraditional health care. Among the worst problems I commonly see with criticism of unconventional therapies is that medical professionals often lump together various natural remedies into one suspect category—something that can also mislead the consumer.

For example, the *Journal of the American College of Obstetrics and Gynecology* (produced by the society to which virtually all obstetricians and gynecologists belong) recently published the experience of a woman who was supposedly taking phytoestrogens (estrogens from plants) and consequently developed endometrial cancer. Most readers of the article would inevitably conclude that these plant estrogens are not safe, that they cause cancer and, in fact, may be even more dangerous than synthetic estrogen.

I was more than a bit skeptical. After a bit of detective work, I discovered that the woman in the article was obese (which put her at high risk for developing uterine cancer), was probably producing excess estrogen because of her excess body fat, and was most likely not ovulating (she was seeking infertility treatments at the time). Remember that failure to ovulate raises the risk of uterine cancer. None of these factors were considered by the article's authors. To top it off, the "phytoestrogens" the woman was taking were in fact black cohosh, vitex (chaste berry) and ginseng, none of which are true phytoestrogens. The authors were obviously unaware of this.

So I have to ask here, when it comes to alternative treatments, can you really trust your physician? If this article represents the knowledge pool of the average doctor, the likely answer is "no."

## A Patient-Doctor Consultation Should Be Just That

Time is another tool that plays into my preventive approach to medicine. As I discuss elsewhere in the book, one of the basic problems plaguing today's health care is the lack of time between a doctor and patient. Very little communication takes place between the two. For my part, however, when a woman comes to me for a consultation, she leaves with an education (whether she wants one or not). I firmly believe that an in-depth, take-as-much-time-as-we-need visit between a doctor and patient can work wonders for preventing all kinds of problems down the road.

I recently saw a woman who was warned by another of my patients to "expect a lecture from Dr. Townsend." It's true. She received my "crash course" on lowering her risk of heart disease, cancer and Alzheimer's disease. We also talked about the merits of genistein, transfer factor, natural progesterone cream and diet changes. After twenty minutes of discussion, she decided to begin a soy-based diet and to try natural progesterone cream. We've since had a couple of follow-up visits—which have involved as much discussion as necessary to answer all her questions and cover her concerns—and her health seems to really have improved. It's during consultations like these that a doctor gets to know his patient. Sadly, most doctors never do.

Another long-forgotten institution that can further disease prevention is the good old-fashioned house call. Virtually obsolete, I believe a home visit can be crucial, especially in rural areas or for home-bound patients. Personally, I love making house calls (especially to patients who live in the country, where I have an excuse to do a little fishing). I remember one woman who left my clinic with a diagnosis of cervical cancer. Because she spoke no English and her fear of the diagnosis, she refused to come back for treatment. So I went to her home, had a heart-to-heart talk about the severity of the problem, and was eventually able to convince her to receive treatment for her cancer.

In discussions with my patients, whether in my office or at their home, I always let them decide if they want to try a new therapy or not. Let me just say that my "unconventional" approaches net an 80 percent positive response from my patients. What physician wouldn't be thrilled with those kinds of numbers? These remarkable results fuel my enthusiasm for preventive medicine. After all, I'm only looking for those things that will ultimately help my patients.

## Time and Money Well Spent

So what power on earth can prompt a person to forgo that double cheeseburger for a turkey on whole-wheat sandwich? Well, education for starters. When I see a patient, whether it's for a "well visit" or a particular problem, I always take time to discuss basic preventive measures—changing eating habits, using a few supplements and exercising—that could help them now and in the future. I frequently hear the same response, however, when it comes to taking supplements: "I just can't afford them." The truth is, you can't afford *not* to. Or, when I say that I'd like to

## Disease Prevention: Are We Doing Enough?

☐ ▨ ■ ■

Considering the measures we're taking to prevent the onslaught of lifestyle-related diseases, it's difficult to ignore numbers like these:

- North America has one of the highest rates of adult cancer. One study found that over three million people have been diagnosed with at least one of twenty-five different cancers within the past five years.
- Cancer rates in women are especially troubling. The *International Journal of Cancer* reported in 2002 that breast cancer is the most common type of cancer diagnosed. Colorectal cancer is the second leading cause of death in both men and women worldwide, followed by cancer of the lung, bladder and stomach in men.
- The World Health Organization projects that cancer deaths will double over the next twenty years. The number of new cancer cases will increase from ten million to twenty million per year, and deaths from six million to twelve million per year.
- The Centers for Disease Control and Prevention report that heart disease killed 709,894 persons in 2000 and remains the number one killer of women (and men, for that matter). Cancer, stroke and chronic lower respiratory system diseases follow as leading causes of death. Meanwhile, cases of Alzheimer's disease are increasing annually.
- Smoking and diet are the principal causes of an estimated three million cancer cases yearly.
- Funding for the U.S. National Cancer Institute's efforts to find a "cure" has increased from $170 million in 1971 to $4.2 billion currently, yet there is still no sign of a real cure.

## Diet: Can It Prevent Alzheimer's Disease?

□ ▨ ▪ ▪

Some studies on diabetes suggest that diet may help prevent Alzheimer's disease. The findings show a correlation between lowered blood sugar and Alzheimer's. In fact, a string of studies presented at a 2002 international Alzheimer's conference in Stockholm—the largest gathering in history to date of Alzheimer's researchers—provide evidence that risk factors for heart disease and related conditions may also play a role in the development of Alzheimer's. Other research indicates that people can reduce their chances of developing Alzheimer's by taking early steps (interpretation: preventive steps) to treat high blood pressure. In addition, the National Institute on Aging and the Erasmus Medical Center recommend a diet high in antioxidants to prevent Alzheimer's.

review their eating habits, I often hear "I'm fine—I eat three meals a day." I can't emphasize enough that changing your lifestyle will inevitably save you money—and hassle—down the road. For example, smoking can cost up to $200 (or more) a month. Imagine applying that same amount to an array of supplements. Investing seventy-five bucks in a good pair of walking shoes (and using them, of course!) could save countless dollars in potential future health costs.

Now don't misunderstand me. The key to health isn't found in handfuls of pills. Nor is it guaranteed by exercising for a half-hour three times a week. And yes, it does take a bit of effort. You have to spend time educating yourself—read books like this one, go to the library, review studies online, insist on talking with your doctor, and so on. But your efforts will be worth it—both in terms of money and health—especially in the long run.

## Doctor Townsend, Please Help Me!

About eight years ago, Susan came to me for severe vaginal pain. It turns out she had vestibulitis, an uncommon problem that makes sexual intercourse difficult, among other things. She was also suffering from chronic bladder infections and generalized muscle pain throughout her body. Incredibly, by the time of our first appointment, Susan had already seen scores of physicians (including psychiatrists) with little success. She had even visited a well-known clinic, starting on the top floor and seeing every doctor on her way down. This little venture cost over $10,000 and left her in worse shape than before she started!

At first I didn't realize her symptoms were really manifestations of fibromyalgia (which was virtually unheard of at that time), so I tried a number of different therapies without success. Some time later, after I figured she might have fibromyalgia, we started to make some progress. I recommended some drastic dietary changes and urged her to begin a basic exercise regimen. I also had her try a product called "Inducer" which contained transfer factor (an immune system boosting supplement discussed in Chapter 16).

Since making these changes, Susan has experienced a dramatic improvement in all of her symptoms. In fact, I would say that she is 95 percent better than when I first saw her. Although she still gets an occasional bladder infection, the rest of her symptoms are essentially gone. I know that Susan's progress is the result of her new diet and exercise habits, as well as her transfer factor supplementation. What about the thousands of dollars worth of drugs prescribed for Susan's condition—who was benefitting from that? Not Susan, but the pharmaceutical companies, of course.

Chapter 5

■ ■ ■ ■

# You Are What You Eat:
# Women, Weight and Wellness

*To lengthen thy life, lessen thy meals.*
*– Benjamin Franklin*

**Nutrition 101 isn't** a course in medical school. Why? Because it's supposedly not important enough to make the curriculum. Medical students have too much to learn and so little time. Physicians are trained to manage a health crisis. They treat disease after the fact—not before. Diet and exercise are considered irrelevant. And even if they were relevant, who would teach these classes? Ironically, the last thing we need is a certified nutritionist telling us to eat "x" servings of meat and "x" pieces of bread per day. That may have been fine in 1950, but today we know better.

Here's a question: What is the most important tidbit of nutrition know-how we should all learn and understand? And the answer: That staying fit, trim and healthy are all by-products of the same dietary prescription. The first thing a medical student should understand is that teaching their patients how to prevent obesity is the same as teaching them how to prevent disease. It's too bad that diet and exercise aren't emphasized during medical training because the same formula that keeps you fit and trim also keeps you healthy. An excess of 80 million people suffer from obesity, and like many conditions, it sports a new, politically correct term—"metabolic disturbance." Unfortunately, the lip service we've given to diet and exercise has done virtually nothing to remedy the problem. In fact, it's worse than ever.

## Food Illiteracy

Why are we so fat? For one, most of us were not taught to eat properly as children. According to one recent study, the physical activity and fat intake of a girl's parents were better predictors of her risk of obesity than her genetic predisposition. Eating has rapidly devolved into a hodgepodge of fast foods, soda pop, snacks and candy—foods that are easily accessible at every corner vending machine or gas station. We let TV commercials tell us how to eat. Simply stated, we eat too many starchy, sugary and fiberless foods. Unfortunately, it's only after illness strikes that people begin to pay attention to their diet. (I'm as guilty of this as anyone else.)

I was born in the era of the Depression and raised in a household that was affected by tight times. My mother chose the most filling and economically practical foods, not necessarily what was the most healthy. A hearty meal would include potatoes, bread and butter, peas, limp green beans, and some kind of meat topped off with gravy made from pan drippings. Desserts consisted of sugar cookies or cake and ice cream. Those types of meals may satisfy hunger, but they also make one fat and sick. Excessive body fat can lead to all kinds of diseases—arteriosclerosis, high blood pressure and even cancer. In fact, if a man's waist measurement is over forty inches (and a woman's is over thirty-six inches), the risk of colon cancer doubles.

# Women and Weight Gain

I once heard a teenage boy say, "Never tell your mom her diet's not working." Unfortunately, many women fail to permanently lower that number on the scale. Take it from me. I've lost about 6,000 pounds in my life and have gained it all back. It's no secret that women gain weight easier than men—one more injustice in a long list of gender inequities. As a gynecologist, I see scores of women struggling in the battle of the bulge. After decades of counseling women on weight, there is no question in my mind that hormone levels impact appetite, food cravings and fat storage. In addition, a woman's genetic makeup greatly affects how she burns calories and stores fat.

# The Estrogen-Insulin Link

Researchers have found that the hormonal flux that occurs prior to a woman's period impacts her blood sugar levels. Estrogen can increase insulin sensitivity and subsequently lower blood sugar. One of the primary effects of low blood sugar is a ravenous craving for sweets or starchy foods—a fact that may explain why many premenstrual women would walk a mile for a chocolate bar. "Sixty percent of women with PMS notice an increased craving for refined carbohydrates, particularly sugar, chocolate, alcohol, white bread, pastries, white rice and noodles," says Susan Lark, a physician and author of the *PMS Self Help Book*. I know that intense carb cravings affect a great deal of my patients with PMS.

Some experts believe that estrogenic drugs (like HRT and birth control pills) also increase carbohydrate intolerance and food cravings as well, which may account for drug-related weight gain. Consequently, women on synthetic estrogen may be at higher risk for obesity, diabetes and heart disease.

To add insult to injury, it appears that the heavier you are, the more susceptible you are to cravings, binge eating and PMS. Why? Because fat cells produce estrogen. Women carrying extra pounds are more prone to insulin resistance as well, which also impacts estrogen levels. For many women, the vicious cycle of carbohydrate cravings and weight gain continues for years since each problem "feeds" the other.

## Is It Really All in Your Head?

What makes a perfectly rational woman attack a bag of potato chips? Hormones! Scores of women tell me that every month their hunger is hijacked by their hormones. Let me emphasize that when estrogen/progesterone levels go awry, carbohydrate cravings can skyrocket out of control. To add insult to injury, women who experience sugar or carbohydrate cravings may also be at higher risk for PMS. I like to call it the "crave and misbehave" syndrome! According to Elizabeth Somer, another physician and author of *A Diet for All Cycles,* cravings for sweets can reach an all-time high just prior to your period, with daily sugar intake rising to 20 teaspoons or more. And the problem is widespread—I estimate that carbohydrate cravings affect 75 percent of my patients.

A new Dutch study confirms another link between estrogen and food cravings. Researchers found that estrogen impacts serotonin activity in the brain. Take a wild guess at what serotonin controls? That's right—appetite and mood. I've seen this phenomenon played out in my patients time and time again. Serotonin is the body's "feel-good" chemical. Low estrogen levels can cause serotonin levels to dip. Carbohydrates stimulate serotonin production, so a woman who experiences a dip in estrogen and serotonin may have an uncontrollable urge to binge on carbohydrate foods. The estrogen/serotonin connection explains

## Insulin Can Be Hazardous to Your Health

☐ ■ ■ ■

According to some studies, women with high insulin levels have an above average risk of developing breast cancer. (Keep in mind that a woman can be slender and still have high insulin levels.) High-carbohydrate foods like cookies, white bread, cakes, and soda are rapidly broken down into glucose (also called high-glycemic foods). Consequently, your pancreas may react by releasing more insulin than necessary to lower blood sugar. In the short term, this can cause blood sugar to drop below normal. Over time, it may cause insulin resistance (which occurs when the body produces plenty of insulin, but cells fail to react to it, causing sugar to stay in the bloodstream). Insulin resistance is considered a major contributor to type II diabetes, obesity, high blood pressure and heart disease. Scientists have recently linked insulin resistance to PMS symptoms as well. A report in the *American Journal of Obstetrics and Gynecology* suggests that synthetic hormone drugs may also contribute to insulin resistance. How many women who take HRT know this?

why doctors often prescribe SSRI (selective serotonin re-uptake inhibitor) drugs like Prozac to treat depression, obesity, eating disorders and PMS. Why did phen-fen promote weight loss? Because it raised serotonin activity, which blunted appetite (especially for carbs). Unfortunately, it could also kill you. The bottom line is that changes in estrogen can increase appetite for carbohydrates that ultimately lead to weight gain.

## The Stress Factor

Stress can also aggravate carb cravings, and estrogen highs and lows certainly contribute to stress. Most women crave carbohydrate-rich comfort foods when they are stressed. This isn't surprising when you consider that carbohydrates stimulate the production of serotonin, a mood-calming neurotransmitter. Continual stress can fuel unrelenting carbohydrate cravings and stimulate the release of cortisol from the adrenal glands. Cortisol negatively impacts insulin levels and stimulates fat storage. Many women tell me they gain weight much more readily when they're stressed, and there's a physiological reason why. The bad news is that the presence of cortisol in the bloodstream encourages the conversion of calories to fat.

Chronic stress can also leave you more prone to illness. A recent study published in a 1999 issue of *Psychosomatic Medicine* found a direct link between periods of prolonged stress and upper respiratory tract infections. And scientists at Carnegie Mellon University in Pittsburgh found that when people with the flu experienced emotional stress, their symptoms worsened.

## Kick Carb Cravings to the Curb

Women can control stress, carbohydrate cravings and weight gain by making a few simple changes, the most important of which is preventing dramatic swings in estrogen levels. This is best accomplished by using my "dynamic duo" of genistein and natural progesterone (see Chapter 8). Equally important are smart eating and regular exercise, which can keep blood sugar levels even. In my opinion, if women steer clear of sweet and starchy foods, they will not only stabilize their blood sugar levels, but they will be less likely to experience the unwanted effects of estrogen excess as well. I know what you're thinking—what can I substitute for salty, crunchy snacks? Take heart. Pepsico is experimenting with chips and crackers made from vegetables like broccoli that are not deep fried. They are also using healthier ingredients like soy and olive oil in their foods. Ultimately, a women is healthiest when she eats a balanced, varied diet that is low in sugar and high in fiber, complex carbohydrates and lean sources of protein.

Keep in mind that vitamin B6 is needed to convert tryptophan to serotonin, so a deficiency can result in low serotonin levels, which in turn can trigger carbohydrate cravings. Interestingly, women with PMS-related carbohydrate cravings are frequently low in vitamin B6 and magnesium. Remember that magnesium is also needed to normalize blood sugar levels, which impact hunger. An added bonus—this nutrient duo also helps with stress management. I tell my patients to take 50 mg of vitamin B6 and 1,000 mg of chelated magnesium daily.

## Diet: Your Number One Priority

If dietary approaches to your health problems don't interest your doctor, you can still make it your primary concern. I cannot emphasize enough how important diet is. Many of my patients resolve their health problems simply by changing the way they eat. It should be the first line of treatment for PMS, fibrocystic breast disease, endometriosis, female cancers, heart disease, etc. It would be even better if doctors taught healthy eating habits in the first place. Unfortunately, many people don't know what good nutrition is. I can tell you that a balanced diet is not holding a cookie in each hand! It's knowing what foods the human body was designed to thrive on and what foods wreak havoc on it.

# Diets Are Duds

A healthy, balanced diet should not be confused with dieting. Although dieting is a quick way to lose a few pounds, it is not a long-term solution. Magic bullet diets or supplements that promise quick weight loss usually only work temporarily and may even be dangerous. As I said before, I have tried many weight-loss diets over the years (even the high-protein variety), but I always gained the weight back. What was my problem? A lack of exercise coupled with lousy eating patterns.

Millions of dollars are spent each year on weight-loss diets, but obesity continues to be a problem in this country. When I was in Europe, I noticed that very few women in Rome and Paris were overweight. Why? Because they walk a lot, they eat breakfast, lunch and dinner at the same time each day, and they don't snack all day long. (Erratic eating patterns can confuse the brain and upset blood sugar levels.)

# The Secret to Permanent Weight Loss

To succeed at weight loss, your diet needs to be "user friendly" for life. Be wary of any weight loss plan that advocates extremes. Dietary changes and a regular exercise program that you can stick with is the key. I discovered (the hard way) that the only way to control weight is to eat right and exercise. Moreover, while you're losing pounds, you'll be gaining a healthier heart. Dean Ornish, a physician and well-known author of *The Life Choice Diet,* was actually able to reverse coronary artery disease in his patients with dietary changes alone. He had them eliminate foods like red meat and reduce dairy and sugar intake. His very successful diet regime also included plenty of fruits, vegetables, beans, soy foods and whole grains. I believe that the most important thing I have done as a physician is to encourage women to change their diets and begin exercising. Those who have taken me seriously have reaped rich rewards.

## The Lean, Mean Asian Equation

When it comes to smart eating, I think we should look to our neighbors in the Far East. Obviously, they have this nutrition thing down. The Asian diet is high in soy, cabbage, legumes and other vegetables. When meat is added to a dish, it is done in moderation, and Asians eat virtually no dairy products. Additionally, the ratio of protein to carbohydrates is much different than the ratio in the typical American diet. Japanese women, for example, routinely eat lots of cabbage, sprouts, garlic and other veggies in dishes where meat plays a minor role.

Clearly, the reason that Japanese women avoid the miseries of PMS and menopause is one hundred percent due to their diet. They are healthier, thinner and consume less food than their American sisters. What they do eat is low in saturated fats and high in bioflavonoids, isoflavones and friendly fatty acids that come primarily from coldwater fish. Moreover, constant snacking—typical in American culture—doesn't exist in Asia. Just look inside a Japanese kitchen pantry. You won't find potato chips, ding dongs, corn chips or candy bars, although the Westernization of Asia with fast foods and soda pop may be changing things. (Interestingly, research shows that Japanese women who adopt American eating habits are much more susceptible to diseases like cancer than women who keep the traditional Asian diet.)

In addition, because the working class in Asia can't afford to buy expensive red meat, they end up living longer and healthier lives than their rich counterparts who consume pounds of red meat and cheese. Sometimes, progress and prosperity propel us backwards. In the middle ages, the king's tables were filled with creamed parsnips, roasted pig and sugar cakes, and nobles who

## High-Protein, Low-Carb Diets: Panacea or Poison?

◻ ▪ ▪ ▪

High-protein, low-carb diets have been around for over twenty-five years. What sets the latest craze apart is that it's been highly marketed. Yes, you do lose weight on these diets, and yes, you can lower your cholesterol levels, but you need to understand why. When you eat nothing but protein, you go into a metabolic state called acidosis, which will temporarily lower your cholesterol count. Why? Because you are in a fat-burning state, which also includes cholesterol burning. Here's the kicker—not all cholesterol is bad for you. Cholesterol is the basic building block for all hormones and is essential for life. And this acidosis state also lowers the "good" kind of cholesterol (HDL).

While you may see some short-term success with a high-protein, low-carbohydrate diet, your chances of sustaining such a diet are extremely slim, so why go on it at all? The euphoria sparked by this kind of dramatic weight loss will be short-lived. In fact, when you begin to eat normally again, you'll probably end up weighing more than you did when you started the diet. My view, which is shared by many other doctors, is that these diets may give you a temporary loss of weight, but they come with a big price tag in terms of health cost.

A diet that prohibits or limits fruits, vegetables and legumes takes away the very foods that keep the immune system vigilant. Consequently, you may not get necessary vitamins and minerals, and may suffer from nutrient deficiencies. You also are probably not getting the adequate fiber for healthy digestion and blood pressure regulation. High-protein diets often emphasize foods high in saturated fat, which if consumed in large amounts raises a person's risk for diabetes, heart disease, stroke and several kinds of cancer. This is madness. Excessive consumption of protein may also lead to kidney or liver disorders and osteoporosis. In short, consuming large amounts of animal protein and restricting complex carbohydrates leaves the body vulnerable to many diseases, which is why organizations like the American Heart Association warn individuals against such diets.

At a recent national seminar comparing the various diets, this question was directed to a well-known proponent of high-protein diets: "Have any studies been done to determine the short- and long-term safety of a high-protein diet?" His answer was that such studies would be too expensive, yet it is estimated that the diet plan he advocates has made over $25 million over the past several years. What do you think is valued most here—your health or your money?

ate such diets groaned all night from attacks of gout. By contrast, a farmer's diet would have consisted of whole-grain breads, legumes, fiber-filled vegetables grown in nutrient-rich soil, meat from grass-fed animals, and so on. You can also be sure that without the kitchen fridge, these people ate only three meals a day and far fewer calories than we do.

Speaking of food portions and calories, Roy Walford, M.D., a UCLA professor and member of the National Academy of Sciences Committee on Aging, has conducted numerous studies showing that lifelong calorie restriction dramatically prolongs life, as well as maintains optimal brain fitness. He is so convinced by the findings that he now fasts at least one day a week.

## The Perils of Animal Protein

Don't ask me "Where's the beef?" because you won't find it at my house. As far as I'm concerned, red meat kills people. It doesn't take a rocket scientist to realize that people who eat lots of fruits and vegetables and little meat are much healthier than those who do it the other way around. The saturated fat found in red meat and dairy products clogs arteries, puts on pounds, adds carcinogens to the body, interferes with hormones and kills brain cells. Even Shakespeare in *Twelfth Night* referred to heavy beef eaters as "dim witted."

Rex Harrison, a well-known movie star, admitted that because he loved the taste of meat, he was a reluctant (but dedicated) vegetarian. That marbly, white fat that makes your steak more expensive, tasty and tender is what's killing you. Most beef cuts contain between 30 and 75 percent fat (most of which is the saturated variety). As good as beef tastes, I consider store-bought red meat a significant health hazard. Commercial beef comes from cattle that are grain fed and kept in a feedlot. It's also very likely that these animals have been injected with hormones and antibiotics. If that isn't bad enough, I recently learned from one of my patients that many feedlots screen manure and re-feed that portion that doesn't fall through the netting back to the cows. That alone is enough to make me a vegetarian!

If you're one of those people who can't live without a little red meat, then fork out a little more money for range-fed (or grass-fed) meat (deer, elk, buffalo and specialty beef). Range-fed cuts are available through specialty stores that can be found on the internet. Even range-fed meat, however, should be eaten infrequently and in small amounts.

## Red Meat Ain't What It Used to Be

Perhaps you're thinking, but what about grandpa? He slaughtered and ate his own beef and lived until he was ninety-two. Well, red meat didn't always have a bad health reputation. Our ancestors ate the kind of game that didn't clog their arteries. You see, animals that graze on the land (deer, elk, buffalo and cows) produce meat that is much leaner and lower in saturated fat. This type of meat protein is infinitely better for the human body than the grain-fed beef cuts that line our grocery store meat counters. Meat from cows fattened in stockyards is full of high-density fatty acids that stick to our arteries. These animals need to go on diets as badly as we do.

The ratio of omega fats found in meat makes a big difference in how they affect the heart. A recent article in the *Journal of Animal Science* reports that the grain-fed beef can have an abnormal ratio of omega-6 fats to omega-3 fats (twenty-to-one). This is not good news because our diets are already high in omega-6 fatty acids and deplorably low in omega-3s. On the other hand, grass-fed or range-fed beef has a three-to-one ratio of omega-6 to omega-3, which is similar to that found in cold-water fish. Moreover, less than 10 percent of fat from range-fed beef is saturated. Remember that your disease risk goes up if the omega6/omega-3 ratio in your diet exceeds four-to-one. It's obvious why primitive peoples who ate wild game had a totally different fat profile than we do.

## The Chicken and the Egg

Even if you've switched from red to white meat, be aware that all white meat is not created equal. Most poultry cuts sold at the grocery store come from chickens that were confined and fed large amounts of corn for fast fattening. Fortunately, some grocery stores are starting to carry meat from free-range chickens that are allowed to scratch and eat vegetables high in omega-3 fats rather than cornmeal. These chickens, though slightly higher in price, can produce meat and eggs with an omega-6/omega-3 ratio of one to five, compared to a grocery store egg of twenty to one. Chickens that have this healthy ratio are also low in saturated fat (less than 2 percent). You can also purchase special low-cholesterol eggs, but if the hen is raised right, the eggs turn out just fine! In a day when hundreds of egg-laying hens are housed in cramped pens, fed high-sugar grains and given fat-promoting hormones, the old saying, "Don't fool around with mother nature" certainly comes to mind.

## Vegetarian Diets: Are They Superior?

Whether we like it or not, humans are basically herbivores, not carnivores. Just look at your teeth. They're designed for grinding food, not tearing flesh. Unfortunately, most of us don't think a meal is complete unless it features a slab of meat—a notion that is costly to our health. Efforts are now underway to educate people about the benefits of consuming less red meat—or at least choosing meat with a lower fat content. Data shows that the healthiest diet is comprised of lots of vegetables, fruits, grains and beans and much less meat and dairy. Vegetarians have superior defenses against free radicals because they consume more fruits and vegetables (high in antioxidants and phytonutrients). Eating a vegetarian-like diet has consistently been linked to lower mortality rates from cancer, heart disease, high blood pressure, stroke and diabetes.

Smart vegetarians get ample amounts of protein from plant sources like beans. Beans are naturally low in fat and fairly high in quality protein, fiber and complex carbohydrates. Raw nuts are also an excellent source of protein. Few people know that beans, whole grains, and a number of seeds and nuts contain essential fatty acids (like omega-3s). Many people mistakenly assume that these fatty acids are only available in meat and fish. Many health-conscious vegetarians eat low-fat yogurt, organic eggs and some fish, and others also avoid white flour and sugar, hydrogenated oils and most dairy products.

Yes, milk does supply the body with calcium and protein, but it also contains the wrong kind of fat. If you have to drink it, choose low-fat or skim milk. Likewise, cheese contains bad fatty acids and is high in fat calories, so if you must eat it, choose low-fat varieties such as mozarella and Swiss. This way you get the protein without the fat.

Don't be fooled into thinking that low-fat foods are always better, however. Just because something is low in fat doesn't mean it's good for you or won't pack on the pounds. Many low-fat and nonfat foods contain a ton of simple carbohydrates. Just look at the food label. Virtually all low-fat foods contain some form of sugar or corn syrup sweeteners. American sugar consumption is already off the scale and may explain the emerging epidemic of type II diabetes among children as well as adults. With smart food choices, a vegetarian diet is perfectly safe for any woman (even pregnant women). However, I do advise strict vegetarians to take a vitamin B2 supplement.

## The Real Skinny on Soy

Of course, we can't discuss the benefits of a vegetarian diet for women without mentioning soy. The benefits of daily soy consumption are continuing to emerge, especially for heart and hormonal health. Scores of books and articles praise the benefits of soy foods, and I'm not about to argue with them. My beef (no pun intended) with many soy diet suggestions is that most of them are doomed to failure. The truth is that very few women can completely adapt to a Japanese-style, soy-rich diet. Dietary changes have to be practical and realistic, or they won't stick and we're right back to square one. Naturally, some diet modifications are better than none at all, but if I expect my patients to eat tofu, edamame (green soybeans) and miso every day, I'm delusional. George Prentice put it well when he said, "What some call health, if purchased by perpetual anxiety about diet, isn't much better than tedious disease."

In any event, I do recommend adding certain "user-friendly" soy foods to your diet. Soy milk, powders and nuts seem to be the most successfully accepted soy additions. The important thing is to choose a good source of soy isoflavones and consume it every-day. (Keep in mind that soy sauce is not a good source of isoflavones, and many processed foods made from soybean con-centrates have insignificant levels of phytoestrogens.) If you're allergic to soy or can't stomach its taste, use an isoflavone sup-plement that contains genistein (soy's most important com-pound). The estrogen-blocking actions of genistein are too important to miss. I discuss genistein supplements in more detail in Chapters 7 and 8.

# Vegetarian Women Could Put Gynecologists out of Business

Let me categorically state that my vegetarian patients don't experience heavy periods, have little or no PMS, and sail through menopause with few if any signs of osteoporosis. The women who include soy in their diets and grow their own produce do even better. They are so healthy that I've been tempted to offer them some meat so they would need me again! These women provide the most dramatic evidence that animal protein and fats negatively impact the female reproductive system.

Two of my soy-loving patients, who I affectionately call the "Soy Sisters," are the healthiest menopausal women I currently have in my practice and probably the healthiest women I've seen period. They both have five children, are physically fit and are in peak health for their age. Their mammograms are clear, and their breast tissue is not dense. They have strong bones and show no evidence of osteoporosis. Their minds are clear, and their memories are sharp. It's a delight to see them whenever they come in for a checkup. These women take no medication whatsoever, and they have an excellent diet and exercise regimen. Do I recommend their diet to other patients? You bet I do.

## The "Soy Sisters" Diet

I asked the Soy Sisters to share the secrets of their very healthy diet with me. Here's what keeps them in such good shape:

***We Do Eat:***
- complex carbohydrates (whole-grain pastas and bread, brown rice, bran muffins, etc.), usually around five servings per day

- about six ounces of protein each day, usually in the form of skinless chicken, turkey, fish, lean pork, egg beaters and lots of soy products (veggie burgers, soy milk and cheese, veggie butter, tofu, soy nuts, soy nut butter, etc.); we also eat a lot of cooked beans and other legumes, which are good protein sources

- three servings of fruit daily (fresh, frozen or canned without sugar); we also eat half a grapefruit every day for breakfast

- lots of vegetables, about four to five servings daily (counting one cup fresh, or one-half cup cooked as one serving), including green salads and cooked vegetables; we also eat sprouts and have our own mixtures of sprouted beans and grains

- a limited amount of dairy products (two servings daily of non-fat or low-fat milk or yogurt); we also use soy milk in cereals and beverages as a substitute for dairy

- three servings of nuts (not roasted or salted) a day, with almonds being our preference, for essential fatty acids (one serving is about 1 tablespoon of chopped almonds, walnuts or pecans)

### We Do Drink:
- eight to ten glasses of water

### We Do Not Eat:
- refined carbohydrates (white flour, sugar, white rice, etc.)
- red meat and whole eggs

### We Never Consume:
- fried foods, soft drinks, alcohol, tea or coffee

### A Typical Menu for the Soy Sisters:

BREAKFAST
1/2 grapefruit
1/2 cup cooked whole-grain cereal or 3/4 cup high-fiber cold cereal
1/2 cup soy milk
1 egg beater

LUNCH
soy burger with soy cheese on two slices of whole-grain bread
salad with nonfat dressing and sprouts
1 serving fruit (usually an apple or apple sauce)

MID-AFTERNOON SNACK
soy nuts and herb tea or
fresh fruit with almonds

DINNER
small baked potato
3 oz. fish or tofu

cooked vegetables
whole-wheat bread or roll with soy butter
fruit or nonfat frozen yogurt for dessert

EVENING SNACK
brown rice with chopped dates or raisins and chopped almonds,
topped with cinnamon and soy milk (yummy!)

(*Note:* We also make various homemade soups using beans, vegetables and textured vegetable protein to enjoy for lunch and dinner; whole-grain breads are also one of our favorites.)

# Eating for Optimal Hormonal Health: One Size Does Fit All

## Eat More Soy Foods

As I said before, it is not realistic to expect every woman to completely adopt an Asian diet, but women can easily include a few servings of "user-friendly" soy foods into their daily diet. The best way to make the switch is to start small and build up. Aim for between thirty to sixty grams of soy protein daily, since anything less than thirty won't give you the health benefits you want. Begin by including one serving of soy milk or tofu each day. If you can't "convert" to either of those choices, try using a soy powder in a fruit smoothie or shake. Eventually, however, you'll need to consume 50 mg of isoflavones each day, which probably can't be met with just one serving of soy.

When you pick up a soy food, look for its protein and isoflavone content. If the label doesn't list the isoflavone content, you can estimate it. Most soy foods contain between 1 and 2 mg of genistein per gram of protein. Look for terms like isolated soy protein, soy protein isolate or textured soy protein.

Like most things, while some soy is good, more is not necessarily better. It's possible to go overboard with soy consumption. I'm aware of some women who became soy "junkies." These women actually developed breast tenderness, experienced abnormal uterine bleeding, and uterine fibroid growth as a result of eating too much soy. Notwithstanding all of its health benefits, if you consume soy in excess, it can cause problems. For most women, however, that won't be a problem. Choose from the following soy foods:

- soy protein concentrate
- soy flour or meal
- soy nuts
- tempeh
- natto
- edamame (green soybeans)
- tofu
- miso
- okara
- soy milk

## Increase Your Intake of Antioxidant-Rich Foods

Eating a diet rich in a variety of plant foods provides the body with much-needed phytonutrients, many of which are marvelous antioxidants. To get the best selection of phytonutrients, vary the color of veggies from day after day. Increase your intake of cruciferous, cancer-fighting vegetables like cauliflower, broccoli, green and red cabbage, and Brussels sprouts. Tomatoes, garlic and numerous kinds of mushrooms are also superior cancer fighters, and grapes, blueberries and cranberries have a powerful antioxidant punch. Green leafy vegetables like romaine, red and green leaf lettuce, Belgian endive, kale, Swiss chard, collards, spinach, dandelion greens and bok choy should be eaten daily.

Carrots, fennel, onions, zucchini, celery and cucumbers are also great choices. Eat potatoes, rice, corn and peas in moderation, however. They're starchy and will put on pounds.

### Fresh Produce: Beauty is Only Skin Deep

Fresh food is an absolute must, but be wary. You can't judge a head of lettuce by its cover. Those gorgeously displayed fruits and vegetables are more often than not picked green and allowed to ripen off the vine. As a result, their nutrient content can be compromised. Moreover, soil depletion is a global problem that has resulted in the lower mineral content of our produce. For example, USDA testing on spinach reveals that it contained 158 mg of iron (per 100 grams) in 1948 compared with a mere 2.7 mg of iron in the same amount of raw spinach today. In other words, today you'd have to eat over twenty bowls of spinach to get the same iron content found in only one bowl in 1948. Even if produce is grown in nutrient-rich soil, if it is stored for a long time, many of its nutrients can be lost.

Surprisingly, some frozen fruits and vegetables may actually be more nutrient-rich than fresh ones. If produce has been rapidly frozen (flash-frozen) and sealed soon after picking, it may surpass fresh food in its phytonutrient array. The bottom line is that we *must* eat lots of fruits and vegetables if we want the best disease protection.

### Legumes Are Essential

Put on a pot of beans! We've already talked about one stellar legume—the soybean—but lentils, split and chick peas, and all kinds of beans fall into the legume category. Legumes are full of fiber, protein and good (complex) carbohydrates. Personally, I think that beans are the perfect food, and their absence from the American diet has significantly contributed to our health demise as a nation. Beans protect the colon and offer an energy source that have no negative side effects like animal protein (i.e. saturated fat). Many civilizations have subsisted on beans and rice or other bean dishes and have maintained excellent health and disease resistance. The high-fiber content of beans also helps to prevent constipation—a problem common to women. And the better your body eliminates waste, the better its ability to detoxify hormones, metabolize food, and so on.

## Nix the Bad Fats and Add the Good Ones

Much of your breast tissue is made up of fat, and the composition of that fat reflects the kind you put in your mouth. You see, not all fats are bad for you, despite what some diet plans would have you think. Fats and oils are either saturated or unsaturated (monounsaturated and polyunsaturated).

In general, saturated fats come from animal sources and hold their shape at room temperature. Tropical oils such as coconut and palm stay partially solid at room temperature but are also considered saturated. Saturated fats have been linked to certain cancers and higher cholesterol levels. The most common types of saturated fats are butter, lard, cheese, milk and red meat.

The term "hydrogenated or partially hydrogenated" refers to fats that have been chemically converted from a liquid state at room temperature into a solid. Margarine and vegetable shortening fall into this category. This process can create dangerous trans-fatty acids. New data suggests that these fats may be even more dangerous to the heart than saturated fats. Who knew?

Unsaturated fats are derived primarily from plants sources and remain liquid at room temperature. Monounsaturated fats are one of the healthiest types of fats. These heart-friendly fats help to reduce levels of LDL (bad) cholesterol and may also offer some cancer protection, especially for breast and colon cancers. Monounsaturated fats are also typically high in vitamin E, an effective antioxidant. Olive oil, avocado, sesame and pumpkin seeds, and nuts like almonds and hazelnuts all contain monounsaturated fats. Polyunsaturated fats, although healthier than saturated fats, should be consumed in moderation. Vegetable oils like safflower, soybean, corn and sunflower oil are polyunsaturated. These fats can lower LDL cholesterol but can negatively affect good (HDL) cholesterol as well.

## A Crash Course in Essential Fatty Acids

Essential fatty acids (EFAs) like omega-3s and omega-6s, which the body cannot produce on its own, are also found in polyunsaturated fats. High levels of omega-6s (found in vegetable oils like corn, safflower and sesame oil) may raise blood pressure and cause heart problems. Unfortunately, these fatty acids are not in short supply in the typical American diet. Consumption of omega-3 fatty acids in the United States, however, is very limited. In fact, daily intake of this valuable fatty acid has fallen to one-sixth of what it was in the 1850s. (Meanwhile, omega-6 consumption has doubled since 1940.)

Most experts argue that omega-3 and omega-6 fatty acids should be consumed in a ratio of at least one-to-three—one omega-3 for every three omega-6s. Unfortunately, the typical American diet has a ratio of up to one-to-twenty, significantly increasing disease risk. Although humans need to consume more omega-6s than omega-3s, too much of a disparity between them can make us sick.

The best sources of omega-3s are flaxseeds and flax oil, pumpkin seeds, walnut oil and oily fish (mackerel, herring, sardines, bluefin tuna, lake trout and salmon). Vegetables like broccoli, spinach, cabbage and Brussels sprouts are also decent sources, if they are eaten regularly. Boosting your omega-3 intake can improve your heart health, reduce stroke risk, regulate blood sugar and aid with weight loss.

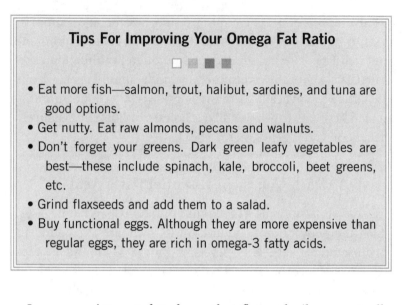

## Tips For Improving Your Omega Fat Ratio

- Eat more fish—salmon, trout, halibut, sardines, and tuna are good options.
- Get nutty. Eat raw almonds, pecans and walnuts.
- Don't forget your greens. Dark green leafy vegetables are best—these include spinach, kale, broccoli, beet greens, etc.
- Grind flaxseeds and add them to a salad.
- Buy functional eggs. Although they are more expensive than regular eggs, they are rich in omega-3 fatty acids.

I was very interested to learn that flaxseed oil may actually decrease the production of dangerous estrogens by blocking their tumor-stimulating actions. According to a 1993 article published in *Clinical Endocrinology Metabolism,* flaxseed enhances progesterone/estradiol ratios during menstruation—a good thing. Women with any estrogen-stimulated cancer need to know this. All women should consume 30 grams of flaxseed oil daily. You can sprinkle flaxseeds on salads or use the oil in dressings, and taking flaxseed oil in supplement form is also an option.

Any woman who is concerned about her hormonal health should boost her omega-3 and monounsaturated fat consumption while limiting the amount of saturated, hydrogenated and omega-6 fats in her diet.

### Switch to Olive Oil

Without question, extra virgin olive oil should be sitting on your kitchen counter. It has been associated with reduced risks for heart disease, breast cancer and colon cancer, and it is delicious on salads and vegetable dishes. It's also great for cooking because of its appealing fatty acid profile. Stored in a cool, dark place, olive oil can last up to six months (or up to a year in the refrigerator).

All olive oils are graded in accordance with the degree of acidity they contain. The best type is cold-pressed extra virgin olive oil, obtained from the first pressing of the olives. It contains only 1 percent acid. (By the way, make sure to read your labels! Fraudulent olive oils are now very common.) Cold-pressed extra virgin olive oil also provides a number of antioxidant phytochemicals that can boost immunity and promote good health if it's not overheated. (For frying, use light olive oils, since heating extra virgin olive oil can reduce its antioxidant content, and darker oils have a stronger taste.) According to a new report in the *European Journal of Clinical Nutrition,* adults who consumed nearly two tablespoons of virgin olive oil daily for one week showed less oxidation of LDL (bad) cholesterol, and higher levels of antioxidant compounds. The *Journal of the National Cancer Institute* also recently reported that extra virgin olive oil reduced the risk of breast and colon cancers by as much as 15 to 20 percent.

Olive oil and garlic are at the heart of the Mediterranean diet and may explain why countries like Italy have lower rates of heart disease. People in Italy and Spain get more than one third of their daily calories from monounsaturated fatty acids (olive oil). Need I say more?

## I Heard It Through the Grapevine

I'm also a great believer in having a glass of red wine with a meal. Wine—in moderation—can help lower cholesterol levels, and it has a relaxing effect. I prefer red wine to white because of its higher levels of proanthocyanidins (a powerful antioxidant).

Be aware that drinking alcohol has been linked to higher incidences of certain cancers (including breast cancer), but I believe the dangers lie in excess consumption of alcoholic beverages coupled with poor eating choices. A small glass of red wine with dinner is good for you.

When processing red wine (not white), grape skins are included in the process of fermentation, which provides the wine's color and adds to its nutrient array. British researchers have isolated compounds in red wine that actually inhibit a protein (endothelin-1) associated with heart disease (the protein causes blood vessel constriction that can impair blood and oxygen flow to the brain). This may explain why some Mediterranean cultures eat saturated fats but have relatively low levels of cardiovascular disease. So the idea that a glass of wine is good for your heart is based on sound biochemistry. Moreover, the impressive antioxidant action of polyphenols puts the "kabosh" on other proteins called tyrosine kinases (involved in cancer cell replication).

Drinking one or two glasses of red wine daily with a meal is now considered heart friendly, although moderation is the key. For those who don't like red wine, a grape skin extract supplement or pure red grape juice may be beneficial. White wine is about 80 percent as beneficial as red, and beer is absolutely worthless. The calorie-laden, carbohydrate-rich beverage does nothing but give you a gut.

## Another Success Story

Joyce came to see me because she heard that I used "alternative medicine." She had all the usual symptoms of estrogen excess—weight gain, bloating, PMS, insomnia, etc. Her exam didn't reveal anything unusual, except that she was a bit overweight. Following a lengthy discussion, she left with a bottle of genistein, some natural progesterone cream and the Soy Sisters' Diet. A month later she

## A Typical Day for the Townsend Family

☐ ▥ ▮ ▮

Many of you may be wondering if I practice what I preach. For curious readers, I have included a sample of what my wife Joan and I like to eat:

**Breakfast**
• High-fiber dry cereal (with good bran content) topped off with one cup of organic wild blueberries and skim milk, and a slice of whole-grain bread

(We occasionally replace this breakfast with an egg substitute, whole-grain muffins, a cup of 50/50 caffeinated/decaffeinated coffee, and at least 8 oz of water.)

**Lunch**
• Water-packed solid tuna salad with lots of sprouts, low-fat mayo and lettuce on whole-grain bread, or
• Salad of broccoli spears, spinach leaves and sliced tomatoes (or spinach, mushrooms, a little avocado and tomatoes) with fresh basil and a small amount of extra virgin olive oil and balsamic vinegar

(Another favorite lunch is a soy bacon, lettuce and tomato sandwich on multigrain bread with sprouts or spinach topped with homegrown tomatoes plus 1 teaspoon of tomato paste.)

**Dinner**
• Steamed cauliflower, broccoli and fresh spinach with lots of tomatoes
• Whole-grain pasta or legumes (We love bean dishes because you don't need animal or dairy sources of protein.)
• Broiled or baked salmon

(For dessert we also like fresh or frozen berries with low-fat dairy topping. There is no need to feel deprived.)

called me to say that she was feeling fantastic and had lost twelve pounds. She put her whole family on the diet and had been enthusiastically distributing it to friends and relatives. Joyce was able to substantially improve the quality of her life without potent drugs. Had she seen another doctor, chances are she would have left with a prescription for a synthetic hormonal drug and that would have been that.

## A Summary of Smart Eating Tips

In short, consume a low-fat, high-fiber diet with plenty of whole grains, fruits (especially berries and grapes) and vegetables, coldwater fish, seeds, nuts and legumes like beans, soy and lentils. Drink at least sixty-four ounces of water each day. If you do eat meat, choose range-fed varieties and free-range poultry and eggs—and keep your serving sizes small. If you like dairy foods, choose low- or no-fat varieties, and use olive oil instead of butter. Stay away from saturated and hydrogenated fats, simple and refined carbohydrates and empty-calorie foods. And of course, cut out tobacco and caffeine entirely.

## Exercise: Just Do It

Abe Lemons once said, "I don't jog because I want to be sick when I die." Well, if you don't move your body, you'll get sick long before you die. Regular physical activity has been proven to prevent obesity, diabetes, depression, cardiovascular and many other diseases. It also increases stamina and endurance, prevents osteoporosis, and boosts circulation to the brain, which discourages memory loss. It also expedites the removal of toxins and waste from the lymphatic system and increases blood flow to the stomach and intestines, which means better digestion.

For years I've heard women say that exercising saved their sanity as well as their figures. Regular exercise helps to ease menstrual cramping, heavy menstrual flow and stress as well as menopausal symptoms stimulated by the ebb and flow of estrogen and progesterone. In fact, several studies have found that women who engage in regular physical activity are less than half as likely to have hot flashes compared with inactive women.

As I mentioned earlier, fat cells make small amounts of estrogen, so carrying even a little extra weight around the midsection can increase estrogen production—a bad thing for women who are already estrogen dominant. Although heavier women may experience less menopausal symptoms because of extra circulating estrogen, they are also at higher risk for breast and uterine cancer. Additionally, young women with weight-induced estrogen dominance are more likely to have menstrual disorders and other health problems.

In some women, exercise alone can ease the symptoms of excess estrogen. And since female metabolism gets slower with age, exercise helps menopausal women maintain their ideal body weight by stoking their fat-burning furnaces. Women entering menopause with strong bones and toned muscles have a great advantage over other women.

Weight-bearing exercise is also very important for women of all ages. Moderate amounts of strength training can actually make women look slimmer and boost their metabolism by creating more lean muscle (more muscle mass means more calories burned—one pound of muscle requires about 35 calories a day, compared with a pound of fat with needs only 1 or 2 calories per day). Most importantly, weight-bearing exercise builds strong bones and is the best way to prevent osteoporosis.

Exercise also impacts brain chemistry, which is often negatively affected by PMS and menopause. One six-month trial published in an issue of *Fertility and Sterility* found that exercise training was associated with less anxiety and depression, regardless of weight loss. And a study in the *Journal of Psychosomatic Research* found that three months of aerobic activity resulted in less PMS-related depression.

With all these advantages, why don't doctors push their female patients to exercise more? I'm sure there are many reasons—perhaps your doctor is inactive himself or maybe he hasn't had much luck getting patients to exercise in the past and has given up. Even if a physician recommends an exercise program to his patients, only four in ten patients actually receive specific advice on putting a plan into action, according to the *American Journal of Preventive Medicine.* How much time does it take to sit down a design a simple exercise plan suited to the needs of a particular patient?

Ultimately, the responsibility is yours. If you make the commitment to get physically fit, tell your doctor what you need, and expect to get it. Unfortunately, instead of firing up the treadmill, too many of us make excuses for our sedentary way of life. One of the most creative excuses I've heard is: "I get plenty of exercise—jumping to conclusions, pushing my luck and dodging deadlines."

## Putting Exercise to the Test

When Lisa came to see me, she was overweight, lethargic, estrogen dominant and had lost interest in sex. She also complained of back pain. I told her that she needed to begin walking every day, starting with at least half a mile per day and working up to about three miles daily. I also suggested that she use weights to build her upper body and begin doing abdominal crunches. She agreed to try, and three months and several pounds later, she came to see me.

The change was dramatic. "Dr. Townsend," she said, "for the first time in years I can see the nice body shape I was born with. I feel fantastic!" Lisa couldn't believe what simple exercise had done for her mental and physical health, not to mention her looks.

# My Exercise Prescription

The exercise advice I give my patients isn't complicated. It's actually very basic stuff that is safe for any healthy adult. (Of course, check with your physician before beginning any exercise program.) First, aim for at least thirty minutes of cardiovascular activity—low to moderate intensity—three to six days a week. Walking, jogging, cycling, swimming, stair climbing, aerobic dance, and the treadmill or Nordic Track are all good aerobic activities. Be sure to incorporate warm-up and cool-down segments into your cardiovascular routine to decrease your chance of injury.

It is also important to include two to three thirty-minute sessions of resistance training or weight-bearing exercise each week. Weight-bearing exercise includes any activity that involves carrying, lifting or pushing a heavy object (or an individual's own body weight). Free weights, exercise balls, resistance cords, and weight machines found at gyms are all good choices. (Walking, jogging, yoga and Pilates are also considered "weight bearing" to some degree, since these activities use a person's own body weight for resistance.) Many women shy away from resistance training for fear that they will bulk up. Keep in mind that you don't need to "pump iron" to build muscle and gain strength. Light weights, such as five- or ten-pound dumbbells, will tone and increase the density of muscles without increasing their size. Don't exclude weight-bearing exercise from your exercise routine. Its bone-protective benefits are too good to miss.

Finally, it's important to stretch for at least ten minutes before you exercise. Increasing your flexibility will help you avoid injury. Warm up by holding each stretch for at least fifteen seconds, and repeat stretches three to five times (alternating sides).

I encourage all my patients to make exercise a top priority. They'll have less hormone-driven symptoms and more energy.

Equally important, they'll live longer and more vibrant lives, and they'll look terrific. In short, they won't be disappointed.

## The Secret to Sticking with an Exercise Routine

Many patients have come to me with a desire to begin and keep an exercise program, but they have been unable to make exercise a lifetime habit. I can sympathize. Before my knees "gave up the ghost," I regularly jogged two to three miles a day, did sit-ups and used weights. As a result, I maintained a reasonably trim body. Unfortunately, spending countless hours on my feet performing surgery destroyed my knees. The good news is that thanks to the miracle of modern medicine, I have a new pair and am currently reestablishing my exercise routine. In fact, I have already lost nearly twenty pounds since my surgery. And keep in mind that after my surgery, I had to learn to walk all over again!

I've heard the plight of many women who start to exercise, then "fall off the wagon." One reason—they try to do too much at once. They set impossible goals and choose routines that don't fit their personalities or schedules. Inevitably they become discouraged and quit after a month or two, which is why I can't emphasize enough the importance of starting slow and building a practical and simple routine.

For this reason, walking is still "numero uno" in my book. It may seem plain jane, but even ten minutes of walking per day can strengthen your heart, elevate your mood and burn a few calories as well. Walk around the block, walk to work, walk upstairs and down, walk your dog—just walk, inside or outside and as often as possible. It's that simple. Even a little movement is better than none at all. If walking doesn't appeal to you, find something that does. My theory on the various and sundry exercise equipment is that most of them work equally well—as long as you use them.

Here are some other tips for making exercise a lifelong habit:

• Make it fun. You won't be able to keep up an exercise habit if it's tedious and exhausting. Do whatever it takes—add music, find a pretty locale or exercise while watching your favorite television show.

• You're more likely to keep exercising if you create an active lifestyle, so pick activities you enjoy where exercise is just a secondary benefit. In other words, if you like swing dancing or mountain hikes, use those interests to help accomplish your goal.

• Choose a convenient time to exercise and make it a habit. Start with a ten-minute walk every day before breakfast or after dinner. After a few weeks, extend your walk by ten or twenty minutes.

• Don't underestimate the importance of variety. If your daily routine becomes boring, try a new time, a new location or a new activity.

• If you miss a day or two, don't despair. Pick up where you left off. And there are plenty of ways to increase your level of physical activity even if you can't make it to the gym or track. Walk the dog or take the kids to the park. Do some gardening or housework. If you are going to the grocery store, park farther away from the entrance to sneak in some extra walking time, or get off the bus a stop or two early and walk the rest of the way to work. The point is to increase your daily activity in any way possible.

• Keep an exercise log, set goals and reward yourself for your accomplishments. It may also help to pair up with someone that you can be accountable to.

• Be patient. It may take time before you see (and feel) results, but it's worth it. In fact, even if you never see an outward improvement, internal benefits are significant and should be the real reason you make time to exercise.

□ ▨ ▩ ▩

# Chapter 6

# Super Supplements

"A man [or woman] too busy to take care of his health is like a mechanic too busy to take care of his tools."

*– Spanish Proverb*

**In June 2002,** the *Journal of the American Medical Association* announced its recommendation that all adults should take vitamin-mineral supplements to help prevent chronic diseases. When I read this, I wanted to exclaim "Hallelujah!" For most people, this announcement was no big deal (in fact, most of you probably never even heard about it). But for those folks within health and medical circles, it was a landmark. To quote directly from the horse's mouth, "Sub-optimal folic acid levels, along with sub-optimal levels of vitamins B6 and B12, are a risk factor for cardiovascular disease, neural tube defects, and colon and breast cancer; low levels of vitamin D contribute to osteopenia and fractures; and low levels of the antioxidant vitamins (vitamins A, E, and C) may increase risk for several chronic diseases, particularly Alzheimer's."

For years, in spite of scores of studies suggesting that a simple multivitamin/mineral supplement was good for you, the medical establishment long held off on officially endorsing the practice. But now, the medical establishment has finally given its seal of approval to basic nutritional supplements—the first step toward preventive health care. The data has been out there for years. We have numerous studies (including a recent Harvard University trial) showing that vitamin E can lower the risk of cardiovascular disease by up to 40 percent. A large body of research supports the notion that acidophilus improves the environment of the gut, which effects our immune function and various other body systems. Other findings indicate that supplementing with various B vitamins can improve or prevent such conditions as heart disease, depression, diabetes and PMS. Calcium prevents osteoporosis. Vitamin C fights free radicals and can help beat the common cold. And the list goes on and on.

Please understand that I'm not talking about having to swallow a handful of pills every day. All that's needed is a little time to investigate and determine which products are best suited to your specific health profile. This chapter won't give you lengthy lists and tables of all the possible supplements you could take, nor will it outline a "25-step plan" to living past 100. Its purpose is simply to convince you of the enormous health value of supplements, and to encourage you to create your own personalized supplement plan that fits your specific needs.

## The Ongoing Supplement Sideshow

In 1996 alone, Americans spent more than $6 billion on dietary supplements, and at the turn of the century, sales had topped $20 billion. In fact, the numbers show that more than half of Americans currently take some kind of nutritional supplement.

In addition, according to a Harvard University study, in 1998 Americans made 629 million visits to alternative practitioners—naturopaths, herbalists, chiropractors, osteopaths, acupuncturists and the like—and paid $12 billion out of their own pockets for those services. This is substantially more than the 385 million visits made to conventional doctors and the $9 billion spent for out-of-pocket costs (and those numbers have in all likelihood increased).

What's behind this incredible trend? Many of my patients explain it this way: "I don't want to use drugs to treat my problems. I want to get well and stay that way." And, many of them are willing to pay "out-of-pocket" for alternative therapies that are rarely covered by insurance plans. The truth is, using supplements will ultimately be cheaper in the long run. Most of these products are safer than drugs and surgical procedures (did you know that up to 5 percent of all heart-bypass patients die on the surgery table?). Moreover, they don't merely mask symptoms or disguise the real causes of health problems. And if you're thinking that you're healthy and don't need supplements, think again. Supplying your body with an ample assortment of vital nutrients will help keep you healthy.

So in the midst of futuristic medical advances like cloning and genetic engineering, an unprecedented swing back to good old-fashioned medicine is in the works. The holistic (or whole-body approach) to healing is regaining its rightful place. People don't want to be treated in "parts" anymore. They want to be viewed as whole beings in which mind, body and spirit are intrinsically interwoven to create either illness or health. In light of the way things are going, I believe that bucking the holistic-medicine movement would be nothing less than professional suicide.

# Using Supplements: A Necessity, Not an Option

You've probably heard that taking vitamins, minerals or other supplements only results in "expensive urine." Your doctor may have even told you that all you need is to eat a "good diet" and you'll be okay. Simply put, these notions are wrong. Now don't misunderstand me. Supplements can't replace a healthful, varied diet. In fact, your diet is the number-one most influential factor in determining your health. But it's becoming more apparent that even the best-designed diet probably won't provide optimal levels of all the nutrients the human body requires. More importantly, while you may live to a ripe old age without supplements, the quality of your health may not be up to snuff. In other terms, you may be alive but have diabetes, osteoporosis, arthritis or heart disease. Scores of studies back the idea that supplementing even a well-rounded diet is a good idea. Thousands of health professionals agree. And the "old-school" medical establishment is finally relenting and recommending that all adults take at least a basic vitamin-mineral supplement daily.

Unquestionably, Americans (and an increasing number of Canadians, Europeans, Asians and folks the world over) eat horribly. There are two principal reasons for this. Our frantic lifestyles don't allow us adequate time to prepare healthful and varied diets. And our food industries have long catered to our convenience-seeking mentality by offering fat-, sugar- and chemical-laden foods at the fast-food drive-thru and on supermarket shelves. Sadly, we often believe the claims plastered on advertising and food labels. Case in point—I'm one-hundred-percent positive that sugar-frosted flakes are *not* "part of a complete and healthy breakfast."

The truth is that eating on the run, choosing sweet, fatty foods as meal replacements, and using caffeine for energy are more the rule than the exception. Unquestionably, the majority of Americans aren't even getting the nutrient levels set by RDA (recommended daily allowances). To make things worse, RDA standards are deplorably low. While the standard now sports a new name, "DRI" (dietary reference intake), it still fails to address worst case health scenarios, where more nutrients are required by the body.

## Are We Really Nutrient Deficient?

☐ ▨ ▧ ▧

Yes. Emerging statistics show that large segments of our population are deficient in one or more nutrients, including B vitamins, chromium, iron, selenium, calcium, magnesium and zinc. A 2003 review of selenium in *Medical Science Monitor* states that while more research is needed, selenium deficiencies are linked to heart disease, reduced immune function, liver dysfunction, and abnormalities in the brain and prostate. It also states that "content of selenium in food depends on the selenium content of the soil where the plants are grown or the animals are raised," and says that different forms of selenium are better utilized by the body than others. This supports the point that we can't completely trust our diet to supply the necessary nutrients.

In the area of cancer alone, deficiencies in vitamins A, C and E have all been connected to an increased risk for the disease. Copper and zinc depletions impact immunity, and low chromium levels are thought to affect rising cholesterol levels and blood sugar disorders. Low potassium levels are connected to an increased risk of high blood pressure and stroke. We know that low magnesium levels can worsen PMS and higher levels of folic acid definitely decrease the risk of birth defects. And calcium depletion is the number one risk factor associated with osteoporosis. Need I say more?

Keep in mind that the "official" nutrition guidelines provided by the various government agencies (the RDAs, DRIs, and Food Pyramid) are widely regarded as inadequate. So, while we think we may be getting enough vitamin C when we consume the recommended 60 mg a day, all we're really getting is the bare minimum needed to ward off scurvy. Most nutrition experts advise taking far more than 60 mg daily—some even as high as 2,000 mg. This scenario is repeated across the board for most nutrients. And it creates a real problem for even health-conscious folks who think they're getting a full array of nutrients. In many cases, the RDA requirements have been cut to the bone.

Finally, these same nutrition standards fail to address each of us as individuals. What I mean is that while there are general rules that apply to human health, each of our bodies may have different needs. For instance, my body may need twice as much selenium as yours to function optimally. Additionally, there are many of us that have increased need of certain nutrients because of any number of "worst-case" factors—such as chronic illness, extreme mental/emotional stress for extended periods, smoking (or living with someone who does), or a toxic environment. For these people, taking nutritional supplements can literally be a lifesaver.

## Women, Supplements and Nutrient Deficiencies

Women are especially prone to nutrient deficiencies, and therefore, more in need of dietary supplements. For one thing, women go on diets far more often than do men, they take birth-control pills (which deplete the body of certain nutrients), they typically lose iron during their periods, and pregnancy can deplete them of calcium, folic acid and other essential nutrients.

It boils down to the idea of "pay now or pay later." For example, we know that if women consume adequate and absorbable amounts of calcium, magnesium and vitamin D in their younger years, their risk of hip fractures drops dramatically later on. Does the old adage "an ounce of prevention is worth a pound of cure" come to mind?

I recently surveyed calcium products at a local health food

## Supplement Savvy

☐ ▪ ▪ ▪

So, what should you do to find out which supplements are best for you? There are a number of things. First, you can get in touch with a reputable naturopath—he or she can provide reliable guidance (don't rely on your medical doctor—they're probably not real familiar with the products). And before you purchase any product, investigate its manufacturer. You can do this online (see the websites below) or by calling the company directly. Frequently, a company's product label will list a toll-free number you call regarding their product profiles and supportive data.

Also, there are a number of books available that evaluate which supplements are legitimate, and even provide reviews for specific products and manufacturers. Finally, you can get on PubMed (sometimes called Medline) and do your own research. PubMed is an extremely large database of scientific studies from most of today's reputable medical and health journals. If a study has been done on a particular supplement, chances are you'll find it there. Here's the web site: http://www.ncbi.nlm.nih.gov/entrez/query.fcgi

A number of other web sites offer unbiased information on the validity of natural compounds and often rate companies for the quality of their products. Some of these include:

www.supplementinfo.org
www.consumerlab.com/news/index.asp
www.uic.edu/pharmacy/research/diet/content/scont_news_grants
www.nmafaculty.org/news/usplaunch.htm
nccam.nih.gov/training/centers

store. A month's supply of a calcium/magnesium mix costs roughly ten dollars (and these are reputable brands). If you project that over five years, you're only paying $500–600 dollars for a sure-fire way to lower your risk of osteoporosis. Compare that to the costs of treating a hip fracture—which could involve initial treatment, major surgery, and rehabilitation—and we're talking tens of thousands of dollars. Moreover, we haven't even touched on the stress, physical suffering, and possible loss of mobility and personal independence that come with such an injury.

Another example—recent studies show that with breast cancer, the aggressive use of nutritional antioxidants, essential fatty acids, and coenzyme Q10 can result in significant remission of the cancer. Additionally, it is well-known that using a multivitamin-mineral daily (especially one containing folic acid) during pregnancy may cut two of the primary causes of infant death—severe birth defects and low-birth weight—by 50 percent! As I was writing this chapter, a news report revealed that supplementing with coenzyme Q10 (coQ10) can reduce the severity of Parkinson's disease. I had to laugh when the network physician advised people with the disease to wait for long-term studies on coQ10 before taking it. This suggestion defies logic. Have you looked at the risks and side effects associated with L-dopa, the drug commonly used to treat Parkinson's? They're frightening—heart problems, vomiting, psychiatric disorders, mental confusion, sleep dysfunction, among many others. I'm not saying that coenzyme Q10 is going to cure Parkinson's. But to advise victims of Parkinson's to wait for long-term studies assuring its safety is absurd. And this is the case with most supplements—compared to drugs, most natural compounds are infinitely safer and have far fewer side effects.

Simply put, a well-designed supplement program, though it may only consist of a few products, can play a vital role in shaping your good health. While supplements can't replace a healthful diet, they are very helpful—maybe even crucial—in providing your body with essential nutrients that it isn't receiving otherwise. Maybe you've never used supplements, or maybe you think they're all hype. Perhaps you're wary of falling prey to a nicely packaged product that is virtually worthless. Don't fear. You can find plenty of quality, science-backed products. And it may take a little effort to decide which supplements you need. But it could make a significant difference in your health.

□ ▓ ■ ▓

# Chapter 7

# A Primer on Phytoestrogens

Discovery consists in seeing what everybody else has seen
and thinking what nobody else has thought.
– *Albert Szent-Gyorgi*

**Diamonds aren't a** girl's best friend—plant estrogens are. *Phyto* is
the Greek word for plant. The term *phytoestrogen* refers to compounds found in certain plants that act as "weak" (mild) estrogens.
They have chemical structures that so closely resemble human
estrogen, they fool the female body. In fact, they exert a distinctly
unique dual action. In premenopausal women, they help to ease a
high-estrogen load, and in aging women, they supplement declining estrogen. For this clever two-fold benefit we must thank Mother
Nature, who in this instance, has really been true to her gender!

## Making Estrogen Safe

If you're looking for a way to safely increase estrogenic action
in your body while simultaneously blocking dangerous estrogens
made by your body, phytoestrogens are for you. Researchers at

the Department of Obstetrics and Gynecology at the University of Bari in Italy, recently reported that phytoestrogens also increase bone density and reduce cholesterol. They endorsed the estrogenic effects of phytoestrogens, describing them as useful in preventing postmenopausal cardiovascular disease as well as osteoporosis. Who knew?

## Smart Plants

You may think that the last place you'd expect a hormone-like substance is in a plant. Their existence, however, is thought to be a plant-protective one. Some botanists believe that these estrogenic chemicals ward off plant-eating predators, much like thorns on a rose bush. Interestingly, if an animal has an appetite for a particular phytoestrogenic plant and keeps eating it, it will eventually become infertile (though you and I don't really have to worry about this potential side effect). You do the math—less plant-eating animals mean more plants. Phytoestrogens also protect plant tissue from oxidative injury, just as they do for human tissue.

Over three hundred plants have been singled out for their phytoestrogen content, but only a few provide what I would call a "superior" source. For example, bean sprouts, sunflower seeds, sesame seeds, rye, and linseeds all contain phytoestrogens, but ounce-for-ounce, soybeans, red clover and an Asian plant called kudzu contain the most isoflavones (the compounds that render the estrogenic effect).

## Getting Back into Balance

The single most important reason women suffer from PMS and other hormone-induced problems is because their estrogen-to-progesterone ratio has become skewed. When estrogen is not properly balanced with progesterone (sometimes called estrogen dominance), it stimulates a variety of feminine discomforts (i.e. bloating, tender breasts, cramps, heavy menstrual flow and fibroids). Plant estrogens help normalize your body's hormonal balancing act by getting out-of-whack ratios back into sync.

The isoflavones found in soy, red clover and kudzu bump potent estrogens off of receptors cells, replacing them with a gentler, kinder version, which reduces estrogen-driven bloating, cramping and mood swings typically seen in PMS.

As previously mentioned, isoflavones are also "smart" enough to exert a mild, safe estrogenic effect for women whose estrogen levels are declining. Some speculate that a consistent intake of isoflavones can keep blood levels of this weak form of estrogen high enough to mitigate some of the unwanted effects of menopause. Chapters 7–9 discuss how to use isoflavones during menopause.

# For Which Conditions Are Phytoestrogens Useful?

Unlike synthetic hormone drugs, phytoestrogens appear to safely balance and support the female reproductive system, making them useful for a number of female maladies that impact the breast and endometrium, as well as menopausal symptoms, premenstrual syndrome (PMS) and osteoporosis. How? Phytoestrogens have the unique ability to compete with human estrogens for tissue receptor sites. By consuming phytoestrogens, a woman can block potentially dangerous human estrogens like estradiol that can predispose her to reproductive and other disorders.

Of equal importance is the fact that phytoestrogens inhibit certain enzymatic reactions involved in the growth of cancerous cells. They also contain an impressive array of other phytonutrients that offer further cellular protection against diseases like cancer. Numerous animal studies provide convincing evidence that the isoflavones found in soy may protect against breast cancer.

## Phytoestrogens and Cancer

A controlled study published in a 1997 edition of *Lancet* assessed the link between phytoestrogen consumption and breast cancer risk. Researchers concluded that a high urinary excretion of phytoestrogens correlated with a reduction in breast cancer risk. Of course, the only way that you can get phytoestrogens in your urine is to consume them.

Phytoestrogens are the nemesis of synthetic hormones found in HRT. Plants with estrogen-like substances are "user friendly" and appear to naturally support the female reproductive system. Traditional HRT does just the opposite. Unlike risky synthetic estrogens, plant estrogens are natural and easily accepted compounds that are swiftly broken down and don't build up in human tissue like artificial hormones. (Remember that the accumulation of hormones in tissues can prompt the formation of tumors.) Because phytoestrogens are rapidly metabolized and excreted, they must be continually consumed to consistently enjoy their health benefits. Out of all estrogenic substances found in nature, isoflavones are the most impressive, and their primary sources are soybeans, red clover and kudzu.

## Red Clover

Although I consider myself a "soy man," red clover is gaining credibility as a good source of phytoestrogens. It contains four isoflavones: genistein, daidzein, biochanin and formentin (however, biochanin and formentin must be converted to genistein or daidzein to be effective). Soy may not have as many isoflavones as red clover, but it is richer in genistein. Still, both soy and red clover provide much-needed isoflavones and offer women vital heart-protective properties.

One reason doctors have been pushing HRT is to decrease a woman's risk of postmenopausal coronary heart disease (the number one killer of women). However, using HRT to prevent heart disease is now openly disputed. In fact, very recent data out of the Women's Health Initiative (WHI) suggests that women with heart disease have a higher risk of more serious heart problems if they take HRT. Furthermore, hormone replacement therapy can predispose you to blood clots or stroke. Chapter 9 discusses HRT and its risks in more detail.

## Red Clover for Coronary Health

In 1998, news wires reported the successful use of a compound extracted from red clover called P-081 to significantly increase HDL (good) cholesterol levels in a group of postmenopausal women. Study findings were presented by Australian gynecologist Dr. Rodney J. Barber at the tenth annual meeting of the North American Menopause Society. The study included fifty women between the ages of fifty and sixty-four. Those who received a 50-mg dose of the supplement over a period of several weeks saw a rise in their HDL (good) cholesterol levels by an average of 28.6 percent. More HDLs mean better heart protection.

Another controlled trial published in the March 1999 issue of the *Journal of Clinical Endocrinology and Metabolism* showed that isoflavones in red clover help to keep large blood vessels pliable—something that may help to prevent heart disease. In a placebo-controlled trial, women who received 80 mg of isoflavones derived from red clover improved the elasticity of their arteries by a remarkable 23 percent.

## Endometriosis and Red Clover

The growth of endometrial tissue (the lining of the uterus) is stimulated by the presence of estrogen. Endometriosis occurs when uterine tissue begins growing in unwanted places within the abdominal cavity. As a result, severe cramping, pelvic pain and even infertility can occur. Most drugs designed to treat endometriosis are potent estrogen blockers that come with significant side effects. If taking isoflavones prompts the body to excrete more estrogen, it only stands to reason that red clover (or soy) supplementation would benefit any woman suffering from endometriosis. When the plant's weaker estrogen form binds to receptor sites, potent human estrogen has no place to park itself and is eliminated in the urine. Less circulating estrogen means less endometrial growth and cramping.

## Boosting Breast Health with Isoflavones

This same beneficial effect can occur in the breasts. Fibrocystic breast disease occurs in approximately 80 percent of premenopausal women and can be stimulated by an estrogen overload. Because phytoestrogens attach to breast tissue instead of human estrogens, the growth of benign cysts is discouraged. Some studies show that isoflavones may help treat fibrocystic breast disease, and dozens of studies show that phytoestrogens actually inhibit breast cancer cell growth in vitro. We'll talk more about that later.

## How to Use Red Clover

If you choose to use red clover as a source of isoflavones, you need to take two 500 mg capsules three times daily at mealtimes. Red clover tea can be made by adding one to three teaspoons of the dried herb to a cup of boiling water and steeping it for ten to

## Are Phytoestrogens Safe?

As mentioned at the beginning of this chapter, animals that eat large quantities of phytoestrogenic plants daily can become sterile. Therefore, consuming extremely high amounts of these plants may pose some health risks. But I can tell you right now that unless you plan on grazing on fields of soy or red clover, there is usually no cause for concern. Using phytoestrogens in infants or children has also raised some eyebrows, although soy-based formulas are considered a safe alternative for babies who are allergic to cow's milk. (Naturally, breast milk trumps them both.)

Some studies suggest that humans possess innate safety mechanisms that protect them from overdosing on phytoestrogens but not from xenoestrogens (environmental estrogens). Researchers discovered that plant varieties don't build up in cells and they exit the body easily, thereby decreasing the chance of any unwanted side effects. Regardless, moderation in all things is wise.

fifteen minutes. You will need to drink three cups daily. Keep in mind that it's more difficult to know how many isoflavones you actually get from teas. As is the case with most natural treatments, you may not see any noticeable difference until you've been on the supplement for three to six weeks. And if you stop, benefits will cease. Isoflavone supplements that have been extracted from plants like soy (genistein, etc.) may offer you a more practical way to make sure you get the amount you need daily.

## The Scoop on Kudzu

Kudzu is a high-climbing, twisty vine that also contains plant estrogens. It has been used by ancient and modern Chinese health practitioners for various female complaints. The kudzu root thrives in shady areas and grows wild along roadsides, in thickets and throughout forests in Asia. The kudzu root is rich in isoflavones, and the Chinese Pharmacopoeia suggests taking nine to fifteen grams of kudzu root per day for various ailments. However, if you're looking for estrogen blockage, genistein found in soy sources may offer women a more practical way to get their isoflavones. If you do purchase kudzu products, make sure that they are pure and standardized.

## "Pseudo" Phytoestrogens

In my view, many plants are mistakenly called phytoestrogens. For this reason, I believe that scores of women are opening their wallets to purchase herbs that will do very little to oppose (or block) estrogen in their bodies. That's what it's all about, folks—reducing the number of estrogen receptor sites that come in contact with the body's own estrogen. (Or in menopausal women, boosting declining estrogen levels with plant estrogens.) In other words, a true phytoestrogen mimics estrogen so well that it fools the body on a cellular level. Only plants rich in isoflavones can do this (red clover, soy and kudzu). All others are suspect.

For example, I believe that black cohosh is a phytoestrogen imposter. Yes, it may have been used by Native Americans to treat menstrual cramps, but it appears only to have some benefit for hot flashes and nothing else. It may also be toxic to the liver, so use it with caution. Chaste berry (*Vitex agnus castus*) is also mistaken for a phytoestrogen. As far as I know, its only true hormonal activity is that it may increase progesterone production.

Dong quai has been used in Asia for various female problems including hot flashes, but I remain somewhat skeptical about its overall effectiveness. I have to go with available data and the experiences of my own patients. For this reason, I have decided that the marriage of genistein from soy and natural progesterone cream offers women the best natural alternative to hormonal drugs available today. (See Chapter 8 for more details on genistein and natural progesterone.)

# Xenoestrogens: Synthetic Hormone Imposters

Naturally occurring plant estrogens and compounds called xenoestrogens are two totally different things. Almost all xenoestrogens originate from an industrial source. For example, compounds like DDT (a once-common insecticide) and PCBs are considered xenoestrogens. Why? Because they also mimic estrogen in the body, but unlike plant compounds, they can cause estrogen-driven cancers in people who are exposed to them. Simply put, these synthetic estrogens are dangerous. Their existence in common household items such as plastic wrap and food storage containers may be linked to malignancies, declining sperm counts and fertility problems. The most significant difference between a plant estrogen and a xenoestrogen is the way the compound breaks down in the body. Xenoestrogens accumulate in human and animal tissue (especially fatty tissue) and can stay there for years. (Phytoestrogens, on the other hand, are rapidly broken down and excreted from the body.) The longer a xenoestrogen stays in breast or prostate tissue, the more likely it will prompt the formation of a cancerous tumor. An added benefit of phytoestrogens is that they can bump dangerous xenoestrogens off of receptor cells.

# Genistein: Phytoestrogen Extraordinaire

Clearly, the soybean offers women the richest source of the most powerful phytoestrogen of all, an isoflavone called genistein. As the subject of scores of studies, it has emerged as an invaluable plant hormone that is completely at home within the human body. It's the genistein content of soy protein that makes it so valuable. Genistein not only acts as an estrogen blocker, it also has numerous anticancer properties, lowers cholesterol and protects the prostate. And it exerts a weak estrogenic effect that can benefit women of all ages. I only wish I had known about its impressive array of therapeutic actions years ago. It could have helped so many of my patients.

Soy is also a great source of genistein-rich protein. As more data emerges about the harmful effects of eating fatty red meat, vegetable protein can play a vital role in the reduction of cancer and heart disease. Unfortunately, most American women look to meat for their primary source of protein, regardless of its health threat. According to an article published in a 2001 issue of the *Journal of Clinical Nutrition,* women who ate diets where animal sources provided two-thirds of their protein had a much higher risk of osteoporosis and hip fractures. On the other hand, when the balance of protein was equal between animal and plants, the risk of osteoporosis and hip fractures was dramatically reduced.

As a gynecologist, I am only beginning to appreciate the health potential of phytoestrogens found in marvelous compounds called isoflavones. Mother Nature knew what she was doing when she provided human beings with plant compounds that protect the body from the ill effects of dangerous hormones, natural or otherwise. Genistein, in combination with natural progesterone, has become the backbone of my treatment program for women today. This dynamic duo is the focus of the next chapter.

□ ▨ ■ ▨

# Chapter 8

# The Dynamic Duo: Genistein and Natural Progesterone

Life is one big long chemical reaction.
*– Unknown*

**Recently, a patient** of mine looked at me and said with a smile, "Dr. Townsend, genistein and progesterone cream saved my life. I could have spared myself years of misery, if I had only known." I consider the combination of genistein and natural progesterone cream to be the most exciting natural cocktail available for women's health. It's that simple. Both of these substances are capable of safely treating hormonal miseries in women of all ages. I found this out after years of medical practice, and now I'm like a squeaky wheel—getting out the word to my patients and colleagues who are smart enough to listen. I call genistein and progesterone "the dynamic duo," and in a time when so many women feel skittish about hormonal drugs, their day has come.

## My Conversion to Genistein

Ironically, it was on a routine visit with another doctor that I met a naturopathic physician who introduced me to both genistein and transfer factor. Learning about these remarkable and relatively unknown natural medicines made me wonder what else was out there. After reviewing the data, I was so impressed that I ordered genistein in supplement form for my own patients. I wanted to try it out. I had looked at data on other natural compounds like *Ginkgo biloba*, echinacea, St. John's wort, feverfew, vitex (chaste berry) and ginseng. Of all the natural compounds I studied, genistein impressed me the most. Why? Because it was backed by the most extensive scientific data.

I was so enthused about the potential of this isoflavone that I presented a talk on genistein to my fellow physicians and (to my surprise) no one booed me out of the hall. That was seven years ago and to date, I've given countless talks on the estrogen-blocking action of genistein, and doctors are much more attentive and curious today—a sign of the times. They also like that I arm myself with bona fide clinical studies. A scientific backbone (or lack thereof) is what makes an alternative compound either credible or quackery. And this is why I hang my hat on only a few natural compounds—because I want real and substantive data.

## Estrogen Dominance: When Estrogen Tips the Scale

Most doctors don't have a clue what estrogen dominance means; this ignorance is probably the result of years of medical indoctrination. Estrogen dominance is nothing more than an imbalance between estrogen and progesterone, or "unopposed" estrogen. When estrogen dominates, it binds with more receptor sites in breast and uterine tissue causing weight gain, heavy periods, sore breasts, bloating, PMS, mood swings, etc. These symptoms can affect premenopausal women of all ages, but they usually appear about fifteen years prior to menopause. I also see the condition in women who aren't ovulating (a scenario that can also be artificially caused by birth control pills). As a result, the uterine lining becomes abnormally thick, causing heavy or irregular bleeding. Too much circulating estrogen can also stimulate cells to multiply in the breast and uterus, increasing the risk of cancer.

The odds are that if you're over thirty-five, you suffer from estrogen dominance. The same is true of women with polycystic ovary disease, who not only have to deal with severe estrogen dominance but also suffer with testosterone issues as well—something that accounts for their excess facial hair, etc. No matter what your estrogen levels are, if they aren't balanced by adequate amounts of progesterone, estrogen will dominate, and that's not good. Symptoms of estrogen dominance include:

• weight gain (fat on hips and thighs)
• heavy menstrual flow or irregular periods
• carbohydrate cravings
• depression
• fatigue
• inability to focus
• thyroid dysfunction
• fibrocystic breasts
• uterine fibroids
• PMS
• loss of libido
• mood swings/depression
• certain types of acne
• breast enlargement and tenderness
• water retention
• headaches
• hypoglycemia
• uterine cramping
• infertility

• inability to maintain a pregnancy
• cold hands/feet
• blood sugar disorders
• increased risk of endometrial (uterine) and breast cancer
• blood clotting, which raises the risk of stroke

Ironically, most doctors prescribe a synthetic estrogen drug to treat the above symptoms (which is the last thing you need!). What you do need is a safe source of progesterone.

So, how can a woman best protect herself from estrogen-stimulated changes in her body? She can use genistein (nature's best estrogen blocker) in combination with natural progesterone cream for added hormonal balance. Let's look at genistein first.

## Go with Genistein

Genistein is a remarkable biochemical loaded with extraordinary properties that, up until now, have been overlooked by the medical community. Let me emphasize—if pharmaceutical companies could genetically engineer genistein or modify it so it could be patented, physicians would be scratching out genistein prescriptions right and left. The potential benefits of genistein are reflected in the abundance of new television and magazine ads that tout soy as a menopause marvel. Without question, it is the genistein content of soy that makes it so valuable. Along with its estrogen-blocking actions, genistein also reduces cholesterol levels and lowers the risk of osteoporosis and prostate cancer.

Over two thousand clinical studies clearly indicate that genistein acts as a desirable weak estrogen in the body. This means that genistein has the unique ability to bind to receptor sites in breast and other tissues that would normally link up with estrogens made by the female body. Consequently, they provide significant protection to vulnerable tissue by fooling the body into thinking that its own estrogen has already been there. In this way, it acts as an "anti-estrogen" for women with an excess of circulating estrogen (also called estrogen dominance). Conversely, genistein can also boost estrogenic effects by stimulating safe estrogenic activity in postmenopausal women. Can you think of a drug with that kind of smarts?

At a time when new research questions the safety and validity of HRT, genistein is a wonderful alternative. Unfortunately, I know few physicians who have taken the time to read the studies on soy as I have. I am convinced, however, that genistein will become an integral part of future gynecologic therapies. I give genistein in capsule form to my patients. I also strongly advise all women to eat more soy foods and to waste no time in doing so. As thousands of women contemplate their risks for developing breast cancer and whether they should take hormone replacement therapy (HRT), understanding the estrogenic properties of soy compounds and how to use them is a vitally important issue.

## Why All the Soy Hype?

Soy became the subject of intense interest after studies surfaced confirming that Asian women have markedly lower incidences of estrogen-related diseases such as breast cancer, PMS and menopausal miseries. The data is compelling—Asian women have breast cancer rates up to *ten times* lower than American women. Moreover, soy-eating Japanese women seem much less vulnerable to PMS and don't even have a word to describe hot flashes. In comparison, American women typically stumble through "the change."

For millennia, the Asian diet has been rich in foods made from the soybean. Soy isoflavones are thought to be responsible for these desirable effects. The typical Asian woman receives 30 to 50

## Watch That Morning Cuppa Joe

□ ■ ■ ■

A recent study suggests that drinking more than two cups of coffee daily may boost estrogen levels in women and could make conditions like endometriosis and breast pain worse. A trial of five hundred women, ages thirty-six to forty-five showed that women who drank the most coffee had higher levels of estradiol (a naturally occurring form of estrogen) during the early follicular phase (days one to five of their menstrual cycle). In addition, it was concluded that caffeine (whether it came from coffee or soda) was linked with higher estrogen levels.

These findings are compelling. Women who consumed at least 500 mg of caffeine daily (equal to four or five cups of coffee) had almost 70 percent more estrogen during their early follicular phase than women who consumed no more than 100 mg of caffeine daily (less than one cup of joe). If you can't give up your coffee, switch to decaf varieties that employ a non-chemical based method of decaffeination. And don't forget to use natural progesterone cream and genistein to block estrogen receptors.

mg of isoflavones per day by eating tofu, miso, tempeh and other soy-based foods. By contrast, American women are lucky to get 2 mg of isoflavones daily, and usually do so from foods where soy protein is used to create a more appealing texture. Realistically, few American women eat adequate amounts of soy, and they probably never will. If you don't consume soy foods every day, you won't get enough genistein to provide continual protection.

Ironically, most of the soybean crop raised in this country is used to feed livestock, and if there's any left over, it's shipped to

Japan where the people appreciate it its nutrition value. It's rather amusing that in America, soy-fed animals may be more hormonally healthy than its citizens.

## Genistein: Tofu in a Pill

I like to refer to genistein as "tofu in a pill." I believe taking genistein in supplement form is the next best thing to eating a diet rich in soy foods. Supplemental genistein is an easy way to make sure you're getting the estrogen-blocking action you need on a daily basis. Now, don't get me wrong. Regularly eating soy foods is the optimal way to get isoflavones in your body (most soy foods contain about 1 to 2 mg of genistein per gram of protein). Unfortunately, it rarely happens.

I've also found that genistein can work just as well as synthetic estrogens and progestins in terms of relieving the symptoms of PMS. I also use it in lieu of HRT whenever a patient is willing. And when symptoms are particularly serious, I use it in combination with very low doses of synthetic estrogen. I don't hesitate to give genistein to my patients who are going through menopause or who have had hysterectomies or breast cancer. The data is compelling—overwhelmingly positive, and I'm in favor of it because it works and it's safe.

### How Much Is Enough?

I like to keep genistein doses comparable with typical Asian consumption, though dosages of genistein vary depending on a woman's specific situation. I usually recommend starting out with 35 mg of genistein per day and 3 to 5 mg of daidzein; a ratio similar to what's naturally found in soy foods. Most isoflavone supplements typically combine the two. Women who suffer from troubling hot flashes or other symptoms may need to up their dosage and add natural progesterone for optimal results. In these cases, I raise the dosage to 70 mg of genistein per day.

## How to Take Genistein

Isoflavone supplements should not be taken with high-fiber meals (especially wheat fiber) or their assimilation may be impaired. Antibiotic therapy may also interfere with absorption. I would also advise any woman on HRT to talk to her doctor about weaning herself off synthetic hormones and onto a natural program with his supervision (naturally, that will depend on their understanding of isoflavones and natural progesterone). Be aware that it may take a couple months to see results with genistein and natural progesterone because unlike potent drugs, natural therapies take longer to work. However, they are infinitely safer.

## Are Genistein Supplements Really Safe?

Every time a woman tells me that someone discouraged her from taking genistein in pill form, I have to shake my head. The logic behind this view is that we don't know the long-term effects of using isolated genistein supplements, so we shouldn't do it. There is also a fear that it might stimulate cell replication. This is where common sense needs to come into play. Overwhelming research backs the positive effects of soy isoflavones for reducing cancer cell proliferation in human studies. Any animal study that shows contrary information should be viewed with caution. Look at the Asian diet—it's virtually brimming with soy. The simple truth is that Asian men and women have much less cancer and heart disease than we do. (I would like to see men take genistein as well for prostate protection and its cholesterol-lowering properties.)

If genistein stimulated estrogen-related symptoms, I'd hear about it. I've recommended genistein in reasonable doses for

## Genistein Enhancers

☐ ▨ ■ ▨

Genistein and other isoflavones are better assimilated in the body when adequate amounts of good bacteria inhabit the large intestine. So using an acidophilus supplement is a good idea. In addition, eating complex carbohydrates and decreasing protein consumption helps to cultivate good micro flora in the bowel.

Some women suffer from severe hot flashes even with high doses of genistein and natural progesterone. In these cases, I add a very low dose of estrogen/estradiol (0.5 mg). Since genistein blocks estrogen receptors, I'm not so concerned about stimulating the uterus or breast tissue with the estradiol. I call this "the best of both worlds," where a woman enjoys the benefits of estrogen and genistein without the downside of either.

Quercitin and curcumin also potentiate the action of genistein. Dr. Barry Goldin's research found that adding curcumin (found in turmeric root) to genistein greatly boosted its antiestrogenic effects. Quercitin, a bioflavonoid and powerful antioxidant has a similar effect. (For more information, see Chapters 8 and 15.)

nearly five hundred of my patients, and not one of them has ever reported breast tenderness or heavier periods. To the contrary—the results have been overwhelmingly positive. In fact, as far as I'm concerned, unlike synthetic hormones, there is no downside to genistein therapy. (Many of my patients gasp when I tell them that a great deal of the estrogen used in HRT therapy comes from the urine of pregnant mares.)

As recently as March 2002, the *Journal of the National Cancer Institute* endorsed soy for its ability to reduce the risk of cancer due to its isoflavone content. Moreover, soy expert Herman Adlercreutz, M.D., of the University of Helsinki has said that there is no evidence that phytoestrogens present in foods like soy initiate or stimulate cancer. You can't convince me that extracting the genistein portion of soy protein and consuming it could be detrimental to anyone's health.

Keep in mind that your body naturally separates isoflavones out of soy and converts some of them into genistein by itself. When you take genistein in pill form, you're just skipping a few steps that would occur naturally in the body anyway. This conversion has been done in the lab instead. If you're sure about the purity of a genistein product and reliability of the company that produces it, then by all means use it.

Undoubtedly, critics will continue to insist that extensive, long-term studies on genistein supplementation are completed before it's recommended. Unfortunately we live in the real world, and no one has yet put up the kind of money required for that kind of research on a product that can't be patented. Make no mistake, if someone could patent genistein as a drug, pharmaceutical companies would be clamoring to fund testing.

## Make Up Your Own Mind

I'm a staunch advocate for safe and effective alternatives to HRT whenever possible, but I let my patients make up their own minds. Yes, I tell them all about genistein, show them the data and leave the decision to them. For example, I don't hesitate to point out the following:

• One Italian study of 104 women conducted in 1996 found that using 76 mg of isoflavones daily from isolated soy protein resulted in 45 percent reduction in hot flashes.

• Other studies conducted at the Bowman Gray School of Medicine in Winston-Salem, North Carolina, found that using soy supplements in fifty-one postmenopausal women resulted in a marked decrease in menopausal symptom, as well as an improvement in blood lipid and blood pressure readings. Adding natural progesterone to the mix worked even better.

# Natural Progesterone: The Forgotten Hormone

The other member of my dynamic duo is natural progesterone. After five years of using natural progesterone, I noticed that many of my patients who were using it did not experience fibrocystic breast disease, uterine fibroid tumors, abnormal bleeding, or osteoporosis. The first to recognize the value of progesterone for infertility was Leon Israel in the 1930's. Unfortunately, his ideas were lost in the subsequent estrogen fray when doctors became fixated on synthetic estrogen as *the* hormone for female health. Clearly, another reason natural progesterone disappeared is because unlike synthetic estrogens and progestins, it can't be patented. Since then, virtually every conventional hormone formula has been designed around estrogen. The notion that progesterone has more hormonal clout than estrogen is shocking, and doctors don't like to be shocked.

# You've Got to Be Kidding

When I was initially introduced to the concept of natural progesterone cream, I was skeptical to say the least. I reviewed Dr. John Lee's book, which read more like a novel to me. The idea that one compound could initiate so many different beneficial effects in the female body was rather far-fetched. I had previously used micronized natural progesterone pills for a patient with PMS and wasn't impressed with the results. Now, someone was telling me that a natural progesterone product administered through the skin really worked. Come on! In time, however, I became a believer.

I already knew that genistein could help with estrogen dominance because it blocked estrogen reception. I found, however, that by itself, genistein was often insufficient to control a severe estrogen overload. The addition of natural progesterone was just what the doctor ordered and prompted dramatic improvement in scores of my patients. I can't tell you how many times I've heard "Your dynamic duo saved my life!" Why doctors aren't actively educating their female patients about this extraordinary pair is beyond me. The marriage of genistein to progesterone is nothing less than a health boon to women of all ages.

## The Disappearing Progesterone Act

American women are failing to produce enough progesterone even at relatively young ages. While their estrogen supply seems adequate, progesterone production is alarmingly low. Technically speaking, a failure during the luteal phase of the menstrual cycle (which normally produces 20 to 30 mg of progesterone per day) is a major cause of infertility, and may explain the rising number of young women who can't conceive. Why the progesterone drought? I have my own theories. The consumption of hormonally fattened meat, exposure to environmental estrogens, poor eating habits, the widespread use of birth control pills, and low antioxidant consumption can impair the ovaries' production of progesterone. I find it interesting that so many women feel their best during pregnancy when they're producing up to 400 mg of progesterone per day, as opposed to the normal 20 mg daily.

Progesterone levels also nosedive during the ten to fifteen

years before menopause. Many women have anovulatory cycles during this time, meaning that they make enough estrogen to promote menstruation, but don't produce progesterone. In other words, they're not ovulating. This scenario sets the stage for estrogen dominance. Using progesterone cream can help prevent the symptoms of PMS and other estrogen-driven conditions. Keep in mind that if you fail to ovulate or are in menopause, you lack progesterone, and you should be replacing it.

## What Is Natural Progesterone?

Natural progesterone (made from wild yam and soybeans) closely resembles the molecular structure of progesterone produced in the female body. Through a series of laboratory steps, extracts from these plants are converted to chemical substances that are virtually identical to the progesterone produced in a woman's ovaries—so much so that the body's progesterone hormone receptors can't tell the difference.

By using a high-quality, natural progesterone cream, the adverse effects of estrogen dominance can be mitigated. Raising progesterone levels has many beneficial effects. As mentioned, the surge of progesterone experienced during pregnancy may explain why estrogen-dominant women feel so great when they're expecting. I think this is particularly true for mood elevation and even libido. Look at all of the advantages of using natural progesterone—they're diametrically opposed to the negative actions of excess circulating estrogen.

## The Pro's of Progesterone

While Dr. Lee's claims about *all* of the benefits of natural progesterone may be excessive, I believe that topical progesterone has real value for women. When progesterone production ceases in a woman's body, all kinds of problems crop up. In addition, we are discovering that a lack of progesterone rather than estrogen plays a much greater role in menopausal symptoms than anyone thought.

During menopause, estrogen levels typically drop to around 60 percent of what they were, and as a result, periods stop. Progesterone levels, on the other hand, dwindle to practically nothing. Progesterone is vital to bone building and the prevention of osteoporosis, so for that reason alone, it should be replaced after menopause. In fact, the ability of natural progesterone to prevent and even reverse bone loss is its greatest attribute. Preliminary research suggests that natural progesterone does indeed build bone mass. Notice that I didn't say it simply prevents bone loss. Natural progesterone appears to stimulate osteoblasts (specific cells found in bone), which in turn lay down bone material if adequate amounts of calcium, magnesium and vitamin D are present. (For more details, refer to Chapter 12). I've found that using it during the early phases of menopause provides the best results.

I should also add that menopause is a perfectly natural event, and many women feel better after their periods cease. For those women who aren't so lucky, however, restoring hormone balance by using the natural progesterone-genistein duo is critical to promoting health and longevity.

## Menstrual Bleeding and Progesterone: Two Case Studies

Cindy suffered from heavy bleeding for nine consecutive months, and I put her on a combination of genistein and progesterone cream. She later reported that the bleeding stopped overnight, and her periods became regular once again. Two years later, her gynecologist remarked to me that I had cheated him out of a hysterectomy. I

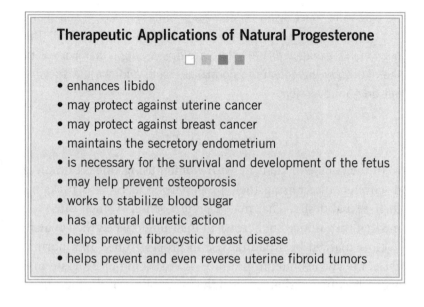

**Therapeutic Applications of Natural Progesterone**

- enhances libido
- may protect against uterine cancer
- may protect against breast cancer
- maintains the secretory endometrium
- is necessary for the survival and development of the fetus
- may help prevent osteoporosis
- works to stabilize blood sugar
- has a natural diuretic action
- helps prevent fibrocystic breast disease
- helps prevent and even reverse uterine fibroid tumors

laughed and offered him my condolences. He said that the impact of genistein and progesterone had profoundly changed Cindy's life, and that I should write up the experience for the *American Journal of Obstetrics and Gynecology.* Once again, I had to laugh and told him that while I had introduced many things into the field of gynecology, the medical profession was not ready to accept this kind of approach. I also reminded him that most gynecologists scoff at the existence of estrogen dominance.

When Marcia came to see me, she was in tears. "I'm still relatively young, but I feel like an old woman. I'm so tired all the time and my periods are getting heavier and lasting longer. To make things worse, I couldn't care less about sex." After chatting with her for a while, it became obvious that Marcia had become yet another victim of estrogen dominance. I told her to quit drinking coffee and soda pop, cut down on red meat, sugar and white flour, exercise and try a course of genistein and natural progesterone cream. She was desperate enough to commit to the program, and we agreed to meet again in six weeks. "I'm here to tell you that I not only feel terrific, I can't keep my hands off my husband! The poor man's exhausted!" All Marcia did was supply her body with the necessary ingredients to normalize itself, and she did so without drug intervention.

## Progesterone and Libido

In the course of chatting with women using "the cream," I've discovered that raising their progesterone levels also perks up their sexual desire. That makes perfect sense. Women often tell me that they notice an increase in their libido when they ovulate (a time marked by a natural rise in progesterone). In a normal cycle, the corpus luteum produces 20 to 30 mg of progesterone every day during what is called the luteal phase of the menstrual cycle.

Perimenopausal women (women in their forties) commonly complain they've lost their desire for sexual intimacy—something I believe is strongly related to low progesterone output. Let me assure you that when your hormones are out of whack, your love life will suffer. When it comes to female hormones, tipping the scales one way or the other is not good. Achieving that precarious balance is what women and their doctors should be aiming for.

## Progestins vs. Natural Progesterone

Progesterone is commonly referred to as the hormone that sustains pregnancy. Over sixty years ago, a progesterone compound was discovered in the sarsaparilla plant (originally used to make old-fashioned root beer). Russell E. Marker isolated a compound from wild yam root, called diosgenin, which would eventually be named a "progesterone precursor." Not only can diosgenin be converted to progesterone in the lab, it can also be turned into a progestin, a synthetic form of progesterone which is commonly used in hormone replacement therapy. Provera belongs to this category of progestin drugs.

In my view, Provera has more side effects than benefits despite the fact that progestins have been aggressively promoted by pharmaceutical companies for years. Sadly, many physicians still mistakenly believe that progestins are the same as progesterone. Nothing could be further from the truth. Their actions in the body are diametrically opposed. For instance, a report in *Gynecological Endocrinology* stated that using natural progesterone is desirable because it poses no risks to liver health, something that is a major concern with progestins. Research also shows that while progestin drugs may damage and constrict arteries, natural progesterone does not. (For more detail, refer to Chapter 9.)

## Provera Pitfalls

Consider the fact that even at levels of 300 to 400 mg (commonly produced during late pregnancy) natural progesterone is still considered safe. On the other hand, taking only a fraction of this amount in the form of a progestin like Provera can cause all kinds of birth defects and health risks to the mother. If you don't believe me, check out the potential side effects of Provera listed in the *Physician's Desk Reference (PDR)*:

- increased risk of birth defects such as heart and limb defects if taken during the first four months of pregnancy
- sudden or partial loss of vision
- possible development of malignant mammary nodules
- unknown consequences if passed in breast milk
- phlebitis, pulmonary embolism and cerebral thrombosis
- fluid retention
- breakthrough bleeding

- depression
- decreased glucose tolerance
- breast tenderness
- rashes

Again, women need to be aware that progestins are powerful hormonal drugs that come with significant risks and side effects, and they are not the same as natural progesterone supplements. Progestins resemble hormones, but are not readily accepted by a woman's body because their artificial chemical structure is identified as something foreign. Moreover, many cardiologists are concerned about progestins because they counteract the beneficial effects that estrogens may have on cholesterol levels. In fact, there is documented evidence that progestins cause coronary vasospasms in some women.

## Should You Walk on the Wild Side?

Natural progesterone creams are usually formulated from wild yam (a root found primarily in Mexico) or a soybean-derived compound. Let me emphasize that creams only containing wild yam will not be powerful enough to stimulate desired reactions in the female body. Yes, the diosgenin content of wild yam is similar to progesterone in its chemical configuration but using it alone has not been proven to raise progesterone levels. In simple terms, there is no proof that wild yam is converted to progesterone after entering the body.

You need to look for progesterone creams that contain USP progesterone, and you'll want to make sure you get between 15 and 20 mg of progesterone daily. USP progesterone is derived from the diosgenin found in Mexican wild yam and soybeans. Through a laboratory process, diosgenin is chemically changed into a compound that is virtually identical to human progesterone and placed in a cream preparation. Some women still

## The PEPI Trial

The National Institutes of Health sponsored the first study—called the PEPI trial—to seriously look at the effectiveness of natural progesterone. This multi-centered, placebo-controlled, double-blind study took place over a three-year period and helped answer many questions about hormone replacement for women. The study involved nearly nine hundred women, and researchers concluded that the combination of estrogen and progesterone did in fact lower women's risk for endometrial cancer. They also found that women who took natural progesterone tended to gain less weight than postmenopausal women taking no hormones at all. More importantly, the study revealed that estrogen combined with natural progesterone provided the best overall protection for women compared to other combined hormone therapies.

insist on using wild yam cream alone, I don't recommend it. In fact, I believe that using a wild yam cream instead of a legitimate natural progesterone cream is an exercise in futility.

### How to Use Natural Progesterone Cream

Natural progesterone is best delivered in a cream form because progesterone doesn't survive the digestive process. Up to 85 percent of an oral dose of natural progesterone is excreted by the liver. But unlike synthetic progestins, natural progesterone is readily utilized in the body without harmful side effects.

Unlike other doctors, I've clarified the application schedule of the cream with a simple recommendation—use it every day. Scores of women have remarked to me that applying the cream to their wrists and directly on their breasts dramatically decreased breast tenderness (another symptom of estrogen excess). Moreover, several of my patients who suffered from fibrocystic disease found that all evidence of the disease disappeared from their mammograms after using the cream. The cream should be applied where the skin is the thinnest and where multiple veins are visible. The wrist, breast and face are the most effective areas for maximum absorption. (In fact, a number of women have delightedly told me that their facial wrinkles diminished following applications of the cream.) The thighs and abdominal wall are poor receptor sites because the skin is tougher, thicker and has more layers of fat with few visible blood vessels. Approximately one-quarter teaspoon of the cream used daily should provide approximately 20 mg of natural progesterone.

### Micronized Progesterone

Typically, the only effective delivery system for natural progesterone was in a topical cream, which allowed the hormone to be absorbed through the skin. Currently, oral micronized progesterone is available by prescription only. It's a form of progesterone that survives digestion and appears to relieve hot flashes, anxiety, depression, sleep problems and sexual function, but it is relatively new and more data is needed. Moreover, in order to get the desired effects, the dosage required has caused undesirable intestinal side effects in some of my patients. I recommend sticking with the cream for now.

## A Match Made in Heaven

I can think of no better supplement duo for women than genistein and natural progesterone cream. I believe that the science to support them is solid, and I've witnessed for myself their wonderful health benefits in so many of my patients. In a time when women are terribly worried about taking hormone replacement therapy, the role of the dynamic duo is more important than ever.

□ ▦ ■ ■

# Chapter 9

# Menopause and Natural Alternatives to HRT

*Formerly, when religion was strong and science weak, men
mistook magic for medicine; now, when science is strong and
religion weak, men mistake medicine for magic.*
*— Thomas Szasz, M.D.*

**In July of 2002,** while I was working on this book, news services
dropped a medical bombshell—researchers in charge of one of
the largest federally funded studies of hormone replacement
therapy concluded that the risks of HRT outweighed its benefits.
The trial was cut short because the data clearly showed that
women taking HRT therapy (Prempro) had a greater risk (almost
30 percent higher) of developing breast cancer, heart attacks,
stroke and blood clots than those who did not take the drugs.

Apparently, fiddling around with Mother Nature by adding
back powerful synthetic hormones to the female body had blown
up in the face of scientists. Last year alone, American druggists
filled over 40 million prescriptions for Premarin and over 20 million for Prempro (the same drug with added progestins).

Women had been told over and over again that HRT would
protect them from heart disease but just the opposite appears to
be the case. They were also promised that HRT would keep their

bones strong and osteoporosis resistant. The reality is that HRT may be beneficial to bone retention, but it doesn't create new bone stores. Moreover, thousands of women were given HRT to remedy their hot flashes, vaginal dryness and other menopausal symptoms. Unfortunately, the cure might be worse than the ailment.

"I will follow that system or regimen which, according to my ability and judgement, I consider for the benefit of my patients, and abstain from whatever is deleterious" is a quote that comes straight from the Hippocratic Oath that all physicians pledge upon their becoming a doctor. When it comes to HRT, that promise may be in jeopardy. Most women take HRT on the advice of their doctors because advertising campaigns make them believe that they have no other viable choices. These women have been led to believe that if they don't take HRT, they are putting their bones and heart at risk.

The FDA has approved scores of HRT drugs over the last half-century without support from large clinical studies to resolve questions about the risks of long-term use. Nor had studies conclusively proved that hormone therapy could prevent heart disease and osteoporosis.

When I heard the announcement that HRT could do more harm than good, I wasn't surprised. (The data has been there for years.) Since the release of the HRT study, my phone's been ringing off the hook with women who want answers. Concerning the synthetic estrogens and progestins that comprise traditional HRT, I tell my patients to get off the damn stuff and use natural supplements! I also tell them that I believe the HRT answer to menopause is all wrong—wrong hormones, wrong formulations, wrong dosages. However, the solution isn't to avoid hormones altogether, but rather to learn how to make estrogen safe. The correct menopausal program can go a long way toward making the transition into menopause as fulfilling, safe and painless as possible.

# Menopause: A New Beginning

Baby boomer women are coming of age—menopausal age. More women than ever before are going through "the change" that signals the end of menstruation and childbearing years. A well-informed doctor will focus on improving the quality of a woman's life postmenopause rather than merely working to extend that life. Women now have a life expectancy of more than eighty years. What this means is that you can expect to live thirty to forty years after menopause. Today, more than ever before, menopause marks a new beginning rather than an ending.

Sadly, for decades many doctors knew less about menopause than their patients did. To illustrate my point, medical textbooks defined this natural transition as a disease (some even referred to it as a "gonadal disorder"). Thankfully, recent years have seen a dramatic shift in how menopause is perceived. Because of breakthroughs in medical science and increased awareness, women entering menopause can now minimize its discomforts and health risks without dread—without sacrificing an ounce of what it means to be a woman.

## Taking the Mystery out of Menopause

Menopause isn't a single event that happens out of the blue. A woman's hormonal landscape actually begins to change up to fifteen years prior to menopause. This transition, called perimenopause, typically starts around the age of forty when changes in menstrual flow and cycle length occur. During this time, a woman's ovaries begin to shrink and she stops ovulating, causing estrogen and progesterone levels to fluctuate. Although there are still enough hormones present to stimulate the growth of the uterine lining, irregularities can cause sporadic periods or abnormal bleeding.

Menopause is characterized by a dramatic drop in estrogen, causing periods to stop completely. A woman is not considered truly menopausal until she has been free of periods (including spotting) for one year. According to the American College of Obstetricians and Gynecologists, fifty-one is the average age of menopause for American women, although natural menopause can occur any time between forty-five and fifty-four. Any woman who has her ovaries removed (an oophorectomy, commonly performed at the same time as a hysterectomy) will experience artificially induced menopause. There are other symptoms of this dramatic estrogen decline, including hot flashes, vaginal dryness, urinary tract problems and short-term memory loss. These can last anywhere from a few months to a few years.

Interestingly, if a woman experiences no side effects from menopause, she may still be at higher risk for heart disease and osteoporosis (two diseases at the center of the HRT controversy). Consequently, every woman going through (or approaching) menopause needs to spend some time educating herself about what to expect—good and bad—so she can make informed decisions about her future. To do this, she needs to be able to separate fact from fiction.

# The Most Common Questions Regarding Menopause

- How can I reduce my risk for heart disease?
- Are HRT or other drugs my only options for dealing with osteoporosis?
- If I take combined HRT to reduce my uterine cancer risk, am I leaving myself vulnerable to breast cancer?
- Without HRT, how can I alleviate hot flashes, vaginal dryness and memory problems?
- Is there another way to stop heavy bleeding without having a

hysterectomy? (For answers to this and other questions about hysterectomy, see Chapter 13.)

• Are soy genistein and natural progesterone cream safe?

• What can I do if I use genistein and natural progesterone but still suffer from hot flashes?

For answers to these questions, read on!

## Estrogen: The Anti-Aging Hormone

Lucille Ball used to say that the secret to staying young was to live honestly, eat slowly and lie about your age. The next best way? Replenish your estrogen and progesterone levels. Don't get me wrong. Just because I'm skeptical about HRT does not mean I don't value using the right kind of estrogen supplementation. I think it's vital for every woman who has had a hysterectomy (and removal of the ovaries) or is going through menopause to understand the pivotal role of estrogen.

Because estrogen has been demonized in recent years, many women have the wrong idea about the hormone. Thanks to oversimplification by the media, estrogen is blamed for countless female health problems. In reality, estrogen imbalance, the presence of environmental estrogens, and the failure to distinguish among different types of estrogens are the real problem.

In addition to its obvious contribution to female development and reproduction, estrogen also influences serotonin levels and fat distribution, protects the heart and bones, impacts sexual desire, and may help prevent the deterioration of brain cells. A lack of estrogen can cause muscle atrophy, shrinkage of the vagina and skeletal weakness. When estrogen levels drop, women can age dramatically. Why? Estrogen helps to maintain collagen in the skin. Without estrogen, wrinkles more easily form. Clearly, women need estrogen. For this reason, safely replenishing estrogen (and progesterone) is crucial to menopausal health. The problem is that not all hormones and their delivery systems are the same. Luckily, there is a way to get the benefits of estrogen safely, even when your body stops producing it.

---

## Cathy's Question

One of my patients is sixty-two and looks forty-two. Cathy eats right, exercises and takes absolutely no supplements or medications of any kind. She has five kids and her uterus is still solid as a rock. To my surprise, Cathy asked me what more she could be doing to maintain her health. I told her that she was doing a great job but that without hormone supplementation, the effects of menopause would eventually take their toll. Cathy decided to follow my suggestions for using genistein, progesterone and vaginal hormone cream, as well as taking extra calcium, magnesium and vitamin D. She is doing better than ever.

# All About HRT

Hormone replacement therapy comes in many forms and in various dosages and is prescribed for differing amounts of time. There are pills, creams, gels, rings, skin patches and injections. Women can also choose estrogen products, progestin products, or a combination of the two. (Keep in mind that progestins are *not* the same as natural progesterone. They are synthetic derivatives of progesterone.) Sometimes a bit of testosterone is added to the HRT mix to enhance libido. The type of HRT prescribed depends on its purpose. For instance, estrogen in vaginal cream or tablet form is often prescribed to treat vaginal dryness or persistent urinary tract infections.

Hormone replacement therapy using a combination of estrogen and progestin came into use after studies suggested that using estrogen alone could increase uterine cancer risk. However, estrogen-only therapy is still incorrectly recommended for women who've had a hysterectomy.

## HRT: Truth or Dare

Initially, doctors started prescribing short-term HRT to alleviate hot flashes and vaginal dryness. When they discovered, however, that a woman's risk for heart disease jumps after menopause, the obvious conclusion was to replace estrogen. Heart disease is the leading cause of death among women, and half of all women over age fifty will suffer from an osteoporosis-related fracture in their lifetime. As a result, researchers began studying HRT to see if it could help with heart disease and bone loss.

Early studies confirmed that estrogen decline is linked to heart and bone problems, so many doctors started recommending that women begin long-term HRT as protection against heart disease and osteoporosis. Nevertheless, other research findings were mixed at best, and for a long time, no large clinical trials were undertaken to truly test the estrogen link to disease or the possible effects of long-term traditional HRT use.

Finally, findings from a study called the "Heart and Estrogen-Progestin Replacement Study"—or HERS—were released in 1998. After following nearly three thousand postmenopausal women with heart disease, researchers determined that women taking combined HRT did not have fewer heart attacks, and their risk for a heart attack actually increased during the first year of use. The study also found an increase in blood clotting. A follow-up study on the HERS participants still found no decrease in heart attacks.

Despite these results, prescriptions for HRT continued to increase. Premarin, the most prescribed drug in America from

1992 through 1999, generated more than \$2 billion in sales for Wyeth Pharmaceuticals in 2001. Plus, more than six million women use Prempro, a combination estrogen-progestin HRT.

So when the National Institutes of Health established the Women's Health Initiative (WHI) in 1991, designed to, among other things, conduct the biggest and most comprehensive study on HRT to date, many HRT-producing companies were thrilled. They were confident that the study would finally prove that all women should use traditional HRT.

## The July 2002 Bombshell

After news spread that one of the WHI's clinical studies on HRT was coming to an abrupt end because of emerging health risks, many women and their doctors were confused. The study, which involved more than sixteen thousand postmenopausal women on Prempro (a combination HRT that contains 0.625 mg of conjugated equine estrogens and 2.5 mg of the progestin medroxyprogesterone acetate), showed that the drug increased breast cancer risk by 26 percent. Users also had 29 percent more heart attacks, 41 percent more strokes and a risk of blood clots four times higher than the placebo group. Ethically speaking, the researchers had no choice but to halt the study, which was originally scheduled to end in 2005. (The other arm of the study involving nearly eleven thousand women using estrogen-only therapy is still underway and will wrap up in 2005 as scheduled.)

Ironically, the study originally touted by pharmaceutical companies as the soon-to-be final proof that HRT protects the heart and bones only raised more questions about its safety. In fact, the American Heart Association now warns postmenopausal women not to use HRT to treat or prevent heart disease. Although estrogen-only HRT appears to positively affect cholesterol, adding progestin to the mix seems to counteract this effect. Some data also suggests that progestins actually cause blood vessels to constrict, reducing oxygen to the heart. You may be thinking, "Okay, so why not take estrogen-only HRT to protect the heart?" Unfortunately, as previously mentioned, this form of HRT raises uterine cancer risk and is used predominantly in women who have had a hysterectomy.

In a press release, Wyeth Pharmaceuticals admitted that combination HRT is not right for every woman, but claimed that it "is the only therapy proven to relieve menopausal symptoms . . . and to prevent osteoporosis in women who have not had a hysterectomy." They also reiterated that for women using combination HRT for only a short time, "the benefits likely outweigh the risks." But even if a woman is not worried about the heart and cancer risks of combined HRT, there are other side effects she may have to deal with, including nausea, abdominal pain, irregular bleeding, breast tenderness, headache, mood changes and hair loss. Progestins can also negatively affect blood sugar in diabetics.

Because women want to ease menopausal symptoms and stop bone loss, they may remain uneasy users of the therapy, but is HRT the only proven way to address these conditions? My answer is a resounding "No!"

## HRT: The Last Word

Approximately 46 percent of American women use traditional HRT. In Japan, the estimate is 6 percent. Of course, each woman must choose for herself whether or not to use HRT, but my patients know where I stand. If I do use hormonal therapies, I recommend the lowest possible effective dose. In the past, estrogen prescriptions were routinely given at 1.25 mg to 2.5 mg per day. These doses didn't take into account issues of estrogen dominance. Today, the common dosage is 0.625 mg.

Additionally, if I do recommend synthetic estrogen, I almost always include it with genistein and natural progesterone cream (the dynamic duo). Many of my patients do just fine using the dynamic duo without any synthetic hormones, but it is possible to take low-dose estrogen-only HRT and the genistein/progesterone combination with minimal risk. For women with severe hot flashes or a higher risk of osteoporosis as well as those who have had their ovaries removed, this "best of both worlds" approach may be their best option.

If you do choose to use HRT, remember that all drugs are not created equal. Be very careful about the form(s) you use and the dosage. I usually discourage women from using "Depo" drugs delivered with an injection or any other delivery system where the hormones stay in your system for weeks or even months. Why? Because if you react badly to them, you're essentially stuck. On the other hand, I prefer vaginal hormone creams. They are safe and effective, and their absorption into the bloodstream is negligible. Above all, carefully look over your medical history and weigh the benefits against the risks before even considering HRT.

## The HRT Headline: One Patient's Reaction

Nancy is fifty-five and stopped taking Prempro "cold turkey" weeks after hearing about its potential risk. Within days after quitting, she started feeling miserable. Nancy's diet included a lot of red meat, she seldom exercised and is a bit "short for her weight." When she came to me for advice, I gave her some diet and exercise suggestions and placed her on a program of genistein, natural progesterone cream, synthetic estrogen (.5 mg a day) and estrogen vaginal cream. After two weeks, Nancy called to tell me that she felt great. She was sleeping well, had no hot flashes and her sex drive was back. She had also started exercising and had changed her diet to include more coldwater fish and less red meat. Nancy's experience is a great illustration of how effective unconventional alternatives to HRT can be.

# Natural Alternatives to HRT

Slowly but surely, more physicians are phasing out conventional HRT in favor of more natural hormone replacement. As you've probably guessed, my recommendation for most women needing hormone therapy include taking the dynamic duo of genistein and natural progesterone and implementing a healthy diet, exercise and lifestyle regimen. So let's review how each of these "unconventional" therapies can help with the disease risks and symptoms that most menopausal women face.

Like synthetic estrogen, plant isoflavones lower cholesterol. However, synthetic estrogen increases the risk of uterine cancer, while isoflavones may protect the uterus and breast from estrogen-stimulated cancer. In addition, natural progesterone protects bones, lowers breast and uterine cancer risk, and reduces fibrocystic breast disease. It may also prevent (or even reverse) signs of aging like skin wrinkles. On the other hand, synthetic progesterone (progestin) carries many disturbing risks. In fact, unlike the body's own progesterone, which is necessary to carry a pregnancy, progestin can actually kill a fetus if taken while a woman is pregnant. (A complete list of side effects associated with progestin can be found in Chapter 8.)

Conventional hormone replacement therapies also often fail to account for women with estrogen dominance. Progesterone levels fall sooner and more drastically than estrogen levels during perimenopause, which causes an imbalance. Even after the ovaries no longer secrete estrogen and progesterone after menopause, they still produce tiny amounts of testosterone that can be converted to estrogen. Couple this with exposure to dangerous environmental "estrogens" (called xenoestrogens) and the result is an estrogen excess.

Estrogen-dominant women have a lot to gain by using genistein and natural progesterone cream instead of conventional HRT. Isoflavones safely boost estrogen levels in menopausal women without causing an excess, and natural progesterone can restore hormone balance without the side effects that accompany progestins.

## Soy Isoflavones: A Safe HRT Alternative for Heart Health

Gregory L. Burke, a medical doctor at the Bowman Gray School of Medicine at Wake Forest University, has studied the use of dietary soy in lieu of HRT. In one double-blind, clinical trial involving fifty-one women given a soy protein for six weeks, researchers noted improvements in menopausal symptoms, blood pressure and cholesterol profiles. Moreover, none of the negative side effects typically associated with HRT occurred.

More research shows the same. According to a study in the *New England Journal of Medicine,* replacing dietary animal protein with soy protein can reduce serum concentrations of total cholesterol and LDL (bad) cholesterol, without interfering with levels of HDL (good) cholesterol. A 1998 Japanese study involving nearly five thousand participants also confirmed that eating soy regularly lowers cholesterol. And in a 1997 issue of *Fertility and Sterility,* data from a clinical study showed that soy isoflavones appear to enhance vascular function and protect the heart. As a result, the FDA has approved soy health claims on food labels associating soy protein with a reduced risk for heart disease.

## Progesterone: The Missing Link

With decades of attention on estrogen for menopause, the role of progesterone has been sorely neglected. As previously mentioned, even menopausal women who have little circulating

---

### Turn to Soy!

□ ■ ■ ■

According to a recent study published in *Obstetrics and Gynecology*, soy supplementation was superior to placebo in reducing the average number of hot flashes during a twenty-four hour period after four, eight and twelve weeks of treatment. By the end of the study, women taking soy experienced a 45 percent reduction in the number of daily hot flashes compared with a 30 percent reduction among placebo-treated women. By the way, my vegetarian soy-eating patients have no hot flashes.

For particularly stubborn cases of hot flashes, you may want to add a very low dose of synthetic estrogen to your routine.

---

estrogen can still suffer from estrogen dominance. Although estrogen production drops during menopause, the creation of progesterone stops altogether.

Without the mitigating effects of progesterone, vulnerable breast and uterine tissues are at risk for cancer. Giving women synthetic estrogen when progesterone is completely absent from their bodies makes matters even worse. In fact, one study found that women low in progesterone are ten times more likely to die from cancer compared with women with normal progesterone levels. Replenishing progesterone levels may be the key to creating the best possible postmenopausal heath scenario for women.

In fact, one double-blind study showed that using a topical preparation of natural progesterone cream led to a hot flash reduction in 83 percent of women using the cream compared with a mere 19 percent improvement in the placebo group. Chapter 8 describes the benefits of natural progesterone in more detail.

## Progesterone and the Osteoporosis Debate

Traditional HRT may not be the bone-protective panacea once thought. In fact, if a woman uses HRT only for a short while to ease menopausal symptoms, she may experience bone loss once she stops. And since traditional long-term HRT comes with many risks, it makes for a risky trade-off if a woman chooses this option to protect her bones.

On the other hand, one of the best reasons to include natural progesterone in your menopausal program is that it may rebuild bone, thereby preventing (or halting the progression of) osteoporosis. When combined with other bone-protective habits—eating a diet rich in calcium and vitamin D, using calcium supplements, engaging in regular weight-bearing exercises (weight training, jogging, tennis), and not drinking or smoking—progesterone is an effective solution to bone loss. For more information on osteoporosis, see Chapter 12.

Using a good natural progesterone cream in combination with genistein supplementation is a fantastic way to lower the disease risk for menopausal and postmenopausal women. And if you are absolutely set on using conventional HRT, estrogen and progesterone creams are also available by prescription and can be formulated at certain "compounding" pharmacies. Now let's take a look at using other HRT alternatives for the most common symptoms of menopause.

# The Famous Hot Flash

Well-known author and columnist Gail Sheehy predicts that "Over the next few years, the boardrooms of America are going to light up with hot flashes." We may laugh at this prospect, but hot flashes are one of the most annoying symptoms of menopause. The sudden rush of heat to the face, arms and neck can last just thirty seconds or up to five minutes, and it really is no fun. A hot flash causes you to feel feverishly hot, sweaty and agitated, followed by a chilling sensation. And because so many episodes seem to occur at night, they can interrupt your sleep. (To top it off, husbands of the hot-flash prone can also suffer when covers are tossed off by their "over-heated" wives.)

Although some men may believe that hot flashes are some-thing women dream up for attention, the condition is grounded in sound biochemistry. Simply put, a hot flash results from a change in the body's thermostat. Body temperature is regulated by a region of the brain called the hypothalamus, which is affect-ed by estrogen levels. When the hypothalamus detects a drop in estrogen, it causes rapid changes in body temperature; hence, the hot flash is born.

Luckily, some menopausal women escape this thermal trial, but most don't. Women who are heavier are actually less prone to hot flashes because their fat stores make estrogen. Now don't get me wrong. This is no reason to carry extra body weight—the risks of obesity far outweigh the benefit of avoiding hot flashes. It is true, however, that if you're slender, your risk of hot flashes goes up.

## Keep Your Cool

If you're having hot flashes, sleep in a cool room and dress in natural fibers. Keeping wet wipes and a battery-operated fan in your purse can also come in handy. Avoid caffeine and alcohol, and don't smoke. Smoking can increase the severity and fre-quency of hot flashes. In addition, research suggests that women who reduce stress levels with meditation and other techniques lessen their hot flash episodes.

## Smart Eats for Menopause

□ ▪ ▪ ▪

I'm all for using soy isoflavones, natural progesterone cream and low-dose estrogen to combat the foibles of menopause, but nothing is as important as what you eat. Diet ultimately determines your hormonal state before and after menopause. The Asian diet is a great example of the positive consequences that come with wise food choices. During the course of my practice, I have seen firsthand what smart eating can do for women, and I have felt the benefits that came from changing my own eating habits. Like it or not, the human body thrives on certain foods, and unfortunately, we usually avoid the very foods we need.

If you are concerned about heart disease, cancer, diabetes and osteoporosis, make diet your number-one priority. Eating for menopause is not very different than eating for optimal health and longevity. It doesn't require a special diet for each symptom or condition. I recommend decreasing or eliminating your intake of red meat and high-fat dairy products. It is also important for you to steer clear of processed and sugary foods, fast food and foods high in saturated or trans fats. Instead, include more whole grains, legumes, fruits and vegetables. Soy foods are a wonderful addition to any diet. Some of the most user friendly sources include tofu, soy milk, tempeh and soy nuts. For a more complete guide on healthy eating habits, see Chapter 5.

Of course, I have already witnessed the positive effects soy has had on me, my wife and many of my patients. The "Soy Sisters" discussed in Chapter 5 are great examples of the health benefits available to those who incorporate soy into their daily diets. And now there are a wide variety of soy foods and soy-based HRT replacements to choose from. I guess that despite pharmaceutical hype, women are becoming less interested in using synthetic hormones.

## The Exercise Answer

☐ ▨ ▪ ▪

It's not surprising that sedentary women are more likely to suffer from moderate to severe hot flashes compared with women who exercise. Many of my patients have remarked that their menopausal symptoms immediately subside after an aerobic workout. Exercise also raises endorphin levels (the happy hormone), keeps weight down and prevents bone loss. What more could you ask for? The choice to exercise is yours, not your doctor's. I'll put it this way—exercise is not optional. For more details on why exercise is crucial, refer to Chapter 4.

### Dawne's Story

Dawne's hot flashes had become unbearable. Her gynecologist gave her a prescription for Prempro to resolve the problem, but after reading about the potential risks associated with the therapy, she stopped using it. She was now searching for a solution.

I recommended that Dawne begin using genistein and natural progesterone cream along with a minimal dose of estradiol (0.5 mg every other day). In a follow-up exam, she told me that she was symptom-free, and it had made a world of difference for her and her husband. Dawne was able to treat the symptoms effectively and safely, without worrying about the potentially dangerous risks associated with conventional HRT.

## Vaginal Dryness and Incontinence

Vaginal dryness is another common complaint of menopausal women. It can make intercourse uncomfortable or downright painful. One of my patients likened it to having sex in the Sahara Desert. Estrogen keeps the vaginal canal moist and its muscles toned. For severe cases, you may try vaginal applications of estrogen (either by cream or tablet) once or twice a week. Such applications also positively affect the muscles of the bladder and rectum. (Atrophy of pelvic tissues due to lack of estrogen often leads to bladder control problems. If you don't want to "depend" on Depends, then use vaginal estrogen to keep your muscles toned.) Even women with a history of breast and uterine cancer can safely use vaginal estrogen applications because the effects are local rather than systemic.

If vaginal applications of estrogen don't relieve the dryness, try using over-the-counter lubricants such as Astroglide. Avoid personal hygiene sprays and douches (as well as perfumed soaps), which can irritate vaginal tissues and promote dryness. Frequent intercourse also helps increase vaginal secretions, and Kegel exercises, which work the muscles of the pelvic floor, reduce incontinence risk. Keep in mind that in order for the Kegel exercises to work, however, they must be done at least one hundred times daily.

In addition, keep in mind that the reason so many postmenopausal women suffer from urinary incontinence is because the muscles that line the vagina and pelvic floor shrink (atrophy). Consequently, sphincter muscles that should hold back the flow of urine, fail to do so. Unfortunately, many women with this problem don't know that using a vaginal estrogen cream coupled with localized exercises (I call it vaginal weight training) can restore a great deal of muscle tone, decreasing episodes of incontinence. It's a simple and effective remedy.

## Case in Point

Fifty-eight-year-old Barbara came to see me because she wanted solutions for severe hot flashes and painful intercourse. She was thin and looked much older than her age, which I attributed to years of smoking. Barbara told me that she had just quit smoking, however, and was also in the process of overhauling her diet. After an examination and lengthy discussion, it was apparent that Barbara was suffering from a lack of estrogen. I emphasized to her the importance of regular exercise and the value of doing Kegel exercises to keep her pelvic muscles toned. I also suggested a program of genistein, natural progesterone cream and vaginal estrogen cream (used twice weekly) to relieve the vaginal dryness which made sex uncomfortable.

After a month, Barbara's pain was gone and her sex life had dramatically improved. Interestingly, she also believed that as a result of the protocol, her face wrinkles had become less noticeable.

## Memory Loss and Mood Swings

If you have difficulty concentrating or remembering details, you can rightfully blame it on menopause. Some of my patients who've had a hysterectomy comment that they regularly fall into a "mental fog." There's a good reason for this. A hysterectomy creates an immediate estrogen crisis that drastically affects brain chemistry. Don't panic. In time, this menopausal effect will lessen. Studies suggesting that drops in estrogen cause permanent mental decline are under attack. In fact, the prevailing notion that conventional HRT prevents Alzheimer's is also in question. Recent studies show that HRT had no effect on cognitive function in women with Alzheimer's disease.

Estrogen also elevates mood, so it only stands to reason that low levels may cause feelings of depression and irritability. Not all women, however, are down in the dumps during menopause. Regular exercise, restful sleep and relaxation techniques can all help fight mood swings. Take comfort in the fact that these mood changes are usually a short-term problem that resolves itself as

## At-a-Glance Alternatives to HRT for Postmenopausal Disorders

There is much you can do to mitigate the negative effects of menopause without resorting to synthetic HRT drugs. The use of specific dietary supplements coupled with lifestyle changes can go a long way to ease menopausal symptoms and prevent serious health disorders associated with menopause. First and foremost on the list should be the two basics—eat a nutritious diet and exercise regularly.

### Osteoporosis
- Engage in regular weight-bearing exercise
- Use natural USP progesterone cream
- Consume isoflavones (soy) daily
- Eat meat sparingly and eat more veggies and fruits
- Take a calcium/magnesium supplement with vitamin D daily
- For more detail, see Chapter 12

### Heart Disease
- Engage in regular aerobic exercise
- Avoid saturated fats (red meat and dairy)
- Eat a diet high in fruits, veggies and fiber
- Eat a daily serving of soy or use genistein supplements
- Don't smoke
- Control your blood sugar and blood pressure
- Consume more omega-3 fatty acids (coldwater fish)

### Hot Flashes
- Dress in 100% cotton clothing (including nightwear and sheets)
- Avoid caffeine
- Eat a daily serving of soy or use genistein supplements

- Use a black cohosh supplement
- Use natural progesterone cream
- Take 400 IU of vitamin E daily
- Don't smoke

**Vaginal Dryness**
- Use a vaginal lubricant (AstroGlide)
- Do not use drying douches or feminine hygiene products
- Use an estrogen-containing vaginal cream or tablet

**Mood or Memory Problems**
- Take an essential fatty acid supplement daily
- Try a course of *Ginkgo biloba* at 180 mg for three months
- Take a B-complex supplement daily
- Exercise regularly to boost circulation and mood

**Insomnia**
- Take your calcium supplement just prior to retiring
- Exercise for twenty minutes early in the day
- Use natural progesterone cream
- Control hot flashes
- Don't eat a large meal after 7:00 PM

the brain adjusts to hormone changes. An extended mood slump should always be checked out by a doctor.

There are other things you can do to help. Try taking an essential fatty acid supplement, which is full of brain-friendly nutrients. And ginkgo, an herb capable of boosting blood flow (oxygen) to brain cells, can improve mental function. Look for ginkgo products labeled "GBE 24/6" and keep in mind that ginkgo must be taken for at least three months to be effective.

Remember that regular exercise also stimulates circulation to the brain and releases hormones called endorphins, which naturally elevate mood. Regular exercise can also raise human growth hormone (HGH) by 25 percent.

## Insomnia

Frequently, women whose estrogen landscape changes as they travel through menopause have trouble with insomnia. I can't tell you how many times I've heard, "Dr. Townsend, I can't get a good night's sleep to save my life." It's obvious that dipping estrogen production affects the brain's sleep center, making a woman more prone to restlessness and anxiety. In addition, night sweats can also interrupt sleep as blankets are thrown off in an attempt to cool down. However, many women who have trouble sleeping during menopause aren't bothered by hot flashes.

Typically these women wake up at two- to three-hour intervals for unknown reasons. Restless leg syndrome can also cause intermittent sleep and seems to worsen in some women after menopause. My advice is to avoid eating after 7:00 in the evening, get off caffeine and alcohol, exercise early in the day, take your calcium/magnesium supplement just prior to retiring (calcium helps calm the nervous system), and use natural progesterone cream and isoflavones to normalize hormone levels. Keeping your bedroom dark and cool is also helpful. Typically, menopause-driven insomnia will resolve itself in time. If your insomnia is severe and consistently lasts for longer than two weeks, talk to your doctor.

## The Last Word

For women and their menopausal miseries, conventional hormone replacement therapy isn't the answer. But neither is doing nothing. One of my goals as a gynecologist has always been to improve the quality of life for my menopausal patients, not to merely extend their lives. So if you're approaching menopause (or going through it), my recommendations are simple but sound. Consider the benefits of eating a healthy diet, engaging in regular exercise and adding the dynamic duo—soy genistein and natural progesterone cream—to your daily regimen. You won't be disappointed.

Chapter 10

□ ▨ ▨ ▨

# Menstrual Cycle Miseries: Common-Sense Answers

Women complain about premenstrual syndrome, but I think of
it as the only time of the month that I can be myself.
– *Roseanne Barr*

**Most women will** (unfortunately) at some time or another have
problems with their menstrual cycle. Those lucky few who aren't
inconvenienced by their periods and can get pregnant without a
hitch probably don't realize how good they have it. Far too many
women suffer from PMS, menstrual pain, irregular or heavy
cycles, and infertility. And I can't tell you how many of my
patients have to plan their lives around (or put their lives on hold
for) their monthly cycle.

Throughout my career I have witnessed great leaps in medical
understanding of the female body, fertility and the menstrual
cycle. There are so many more options available for women now
than were available for their mothers. Still, many women are not
aware of nondrug options for treating problems associated with
their period. Others would like to try something different but cannot get their doctor to prescribe complementary treatments. This
chapter is for these women. I have successfully treated hundreds of

women with menstrual disorders without using potent drugs, and I want to share their health secrets with you.

## PMS: The Birth of a Syndrome

First described in 1931 as a "state of unbearable tension," premenstrual syndrome wasn't recognized as a legitimate medical disorder for decades. To add insult to injury, women who suffered from symptoms related to their periods were lumped together in a catch-all syndrome called PMS. That disorder was defined as a "cluster" of physical and emotional symptoms triggered by the menstrual cycle. Statistics tell us that nearly two out of five women ages fourteen to fifty experience some degree of PMS one to two weeks before their period, and 10 percent of these women have symptoms severe enough to interrupt their routines.

What causes PMS? Doctors know that hormonal imbalances (i.e. estrogen dominance) and faulty serotonin production are involved. That's why hormones and antidepressants (like Prozac, Paxil or other SSRIs) are often prescribed for PMS. Researchers have also linked the stress hormone cortisol to menstrual irregularities. New information, however, suggests that there is much more at play. Personality, age, diet, genetics and a woman's own specific hormonal signature all determine her individual "brand" of PMS.

## Garden Variety PMS: The Most Common Symptoms

"Dr. Townsend, my fuse gets so short a few days before my period that my family goes into hiding," a patient once complained to me. For other patients, water retention and depression are the most common effects of PMS. The estrogen-progesterone see-saw can trigger all kinds of negative reactions. Adding variables like stress, faulty nutrition and birth control pills can make symptoms even more severe. Every woman's body reacts differently to cyclic changes—no two are exactly alike. Caffeine and sugar consumption can also make PMS worse, while salt is often the culprit.

Keep in mind that an ailment you suffer from all month long that worsens in the days prior to your period is not a true symptom of PMS. Conditions like chronic asthma, joint pain and migraines can flare up around your menstrual cycle. Additionally, you may become more prone to colds and sore throats. The reason? Estrogen fluctuations affect DHEA and interleukin levels in the female immune system, making women more susceptible to infections and inflammatory flare-ups.

Many women with PMS also complain of menstrual cramps and lower back pain before and during their periods. Menstrual pain (dysmenorrhea) is not commonly considered a symptom of PMS because it can be caused by other conditions, including pelvic inflammatory disease (PID), endometriosis, fibroids and ovarian cysts. Some doctors even consider menstrual pain in healthy women to be a perfectly normal condition. I've found, however, that women who suffer from painful periods without any known cause can be helped.

More than 150 symptoms have been attributed to PMS. Of course, the symptoms and their severity will vary from woman to woman, but below is a list of the most common premenstrual complaints I receive from my patients:

• acne
• anxiety
• bloating/water retention
• breast tenderness and swelling
• changes in sleeping patterns

- depression
- fatigue/inability to concentrate
- food cravings (especially for carbohydrates and sweets)
- headaches
- irritability
- low libido
- mood swings
- weight gain

## Cortisol: The Stress Connection

Women often ask me, "Does stress make PMS worse or do I feel stressed because I'm premenstrual?" I think it's a little bit of both. Stress and PMS seem to have a reciprocal relationship. Stress increases the release of a hormone called cortisol, which can inhibit the bonding of progesterone to receptor cells. Therefore, if a woman is chronically stressed, the effects of cortisol may cause a hormonal imbalance by interfering with her progesterone levels.

Regardless, all women with PMS emphatically declare that their stress levels skyrocket in the days just prior to their menstrual period. High estrogen levels coupled with low progesterone levels can also cause mood fluctuations. When this happens, a woman feels edgy and short tempered until her period begins. Remember that cortisol is not the only factor that can disrupt hormone levels. Lack of sleep, poor diets or even a B vitamin deficiency can be to blame. Interestingly, vitamin B6 reduces blood levels of estrogen and increases progesterone levels.

## Mood Swings and Depression

Vitamin B6 also supports brain function, as does magnesium. Deficiencies of either nutrient can trigger mood swings. Some of my patients get so blue prior to their period that they can't get out of bed. These women experience crying spells, confusion, feelings of extreme isolation and sometimes thoughts of suicide. Their PMS-driven emotions can range from mild melancholia to severe withdrawal. I have one patient who always knows when her period is about to begin because she feels like running away from home. Many others complain of nervousness, irritability and insomnia. Women with severe emotional and behavioral symptoms may have premenstrual dysphoric disorder (PMDD), which is thought to affect 3–8 percent of all women. Estrogen dominance may also play a role in their depression (estrogen is a nervous system stimulant), but elevated levels of adrenal hormones (androgens) can negatively impact serotonin production in the brain, sparking a depressive episode. The emotional way a woman handles her hormonal ups and downs also depends on her age. The fact is that what we call "mood" is not just a state of being but rather a series of physiological events throughout the body that impact the brain.

# Increased Hunger and Carbohydrate Cravings

Estrogen not only affects brain chemistry, it also influences the brain's "appestat." Many of my patients crave salty, starchy or fatty foods in the days before their period. For instance, a drop in serotonin can trigger a carbohydrate craving (carbohydrates are mood enhancers). However, binging on carbohydrates causes blood sugar levels to spike, prompting the body to release too much insulin. (In some women, salt can also overstimulate insulin production, contributing to unstable blood sugar levels.) Blood sugar then falls in response to excessive amounts of insulin, negatively affecting mood and triggering another craving. And the cycle continues. In other words, an estrogen-dominant, premenstrual woman craves carbohydrates because her brain chemistry tells her to.

Many women also have intense cravings for chocolate. One of my patients said she'd walk a mile for chocolate! This isn't surprising when you consider that chocolate is naturally rich in phenylethylamine, a natural antidepressant containing caffeine and magnesium. Magnesium depletion is common in women with PMS, so chocolate cravings may actually be your body's attempt to tell you something. (Taking supplemental magnesium can also improve your ability to tolerate carbohydrates and sugar.)

## When the Shoe Doesn't Fit

It's not unusual for a woman with PMS to gain three pounds or more before her period. Her hands and feet may swell, her breasts may become tender, and her abdomen can feel bloated and extremely uncomfortable. Why? During an estrogen spike, serum aldosterone levels can increase, causing tissues to retain fluid, and dopamine levels may dip, impairing the kidneys' ability to deal with water and sodium. To make things worse, certain prostaglandin hormones, which aggravate menstrual cramps, can also contribute to water retention.

If you battle bloating, sharply reduce your salt and soda pop intake. Eat no more than 3 grams of salt daily, and avoid caffeine and nicotine entirely. Vitamin B6 and vitamin E help suppress the production of aldosterone, resulting in the more efficient cleaning of fluid from the body. Vitamin E also reduces breast swelling and pain. For sore breasts, I also strongly recommend rubbing natural progesterone cream directly on them. Many women comment that within hours of doing so, the tenderness subsides.

# Cramps, Cramps and More Cramps

Countless women experience cramping before and during their periods. They also sometimes suffer from lower back or inner thigh pain, diarrhea, nausea and even vomiting. In fact, more than half of menstruating women suffer from painful periods, and 10 to 15 percent experience pain severe enough to interfere with their daily activities and require medication.

There are two possible causes for cramping in otherwise healthy women—the presence of menstrual clots and the action of prostaglandins (pain-related chemicals). "Clot cramps" are the result of the build-up of small blood clots within the uterus that are expelled by the muscular contraction of the organ. Chemical culprits called prostaglandins cause uterine spasms and pain. Ibuprofen or acetaminophen is often prescribed to inhibit the actions of prostaglandins, but to be effective they must be taken at the first sign of cramping. Heating pads are also helpful. Women with chronic and severe cases of cramps are often prescribed narcotics or oral contraceptives. I've found that diet, exercise and supplement therapy can help mitigate menstrual pain. Natural progesterone cream is particularly useful, and I like to add 200 mg of niacin daily. Reducing stress levels is also crucial.

Before beginning any self-treatment for cramps, see your doctor, especially if you experience sudden cramping. In some women, cramps may be the result of other problems, such as fibroids, cysts, pelvic inflammatory disease (PID), IUD use or endometriosis. If you are pregnant and feel any cramping, see your doctor immediately.

# The PMS Solution

While there's no "magic bullet" for the miseries of PMS, you can do plenty to ease its symptoms. It's important to understand that PMS is a multi-faceted disorder and is different for every woman. Regardless of your symptoms, however, every woman who suffers from PMS should be using genistein and natural progesterone cream. These two supplements offer the best natural solutions for PMS.

More importantly, every woman needs to understand that her food choices can dramatically impact her hormonal symptoms. I told one of my patients with severe PMS to try genistein and natural progesterone cream, and to change her diet as well. Guess what? The positive impact of better food choices was so dramatic, she didn't need to use the supplements! Her PMS was all but gone, and all she did was cut down on saturated fats (meats, dairy, etc.), limit her sugar and salt intake, and emphasize fruits, vegetables and legumes (beans). She also added the exercise card. It was that simple. An overhaul of her diet basically cured her of PMS.

My vegetarian patients seldom complain of PMS or any other symptoms linked to excess estrogen. That's why I recommend starting with your diet, adding appropriate supplements (genistein, progesterone and a good antioxidant) and exercising regularly for several cycles. Regular aerobic exercise fights all types of PMS. In a 1994 study reported in the *Journal of Psychosomatic Research,* researchers compared ninety-seven women who exercised regularly to 159 who did not. The exercise group had less PMS-related mood slumps, behavioral changes, and pain.

Taking a daily dose of calcium and magnesium can also help chase away the PMS demons. Studies show that regular supplementation may help relieve depression, mood swings, headaches, irritability, and other PMS-related symptoms. In a 1998 study published in the *American Journal of Obstetrics and Gynecology,* nearly 500 women suffering from moderate to severe PMS taking two 750 mg tablets of calcium carbonate twice a day for three months reduced overall severity of symptoms by 50 percent, compared with only 30 percent for those taking a placebo. Another study of forty women from the University of Reading in the U.K. found that those suffering from PMS-related symptoms of fluid retention (bloating, weight gain, swollen arms, breast tenderness) might benefit from taking 200 mg of magnesium oxide daily. After two menstrual cycles, those taking the magnesium had a significant reduction of symptoms compared with those taking a placebo. I prefer calcium citrate to carbonate, although some supplements include both. Make sure you always take calcium with chelated magnesium and vitamin D.

After you've made dietary changes and used the supplements discussed, assess your hormonal landscape. Keeping a calendar or diary of daily symptoms and treatments may help. My experience supports the view that if you do these things, chances are your PMS will become a thing of the past.

### Trudy's Terrible Trial

Trudy, a twenty-six-year-old mother of one, was referred to me because of an abnormal Pap smear. Although the cervical problem turned out to be nothing, her husband was on the verge of ending their marriage because he could no longer cope with her extreme PMS. She said that during the week prior to her period, she could not control her temper and avoided all sexual contact. We discussed diet and exercise, and she agreed to try genistein and natural progesterone cream. Three months later, she told me that her marriage was once again on solid footing, and her PMS symptoms were minimal. I was so impressed by her turnaround, I asked her to return in three months to see how she was progressing. Trudy told me in her follow-up exam that her husband couldn't keep up with her newfound sex drive, and she felt fantastic!

## Endometriosis: Menstruation Gone Awry

Until recently, many endometriosis patients were written off by doctors as neurotic or overly sensitive to pain, and treatments commonly included tranquilizers or hysterectomies. Research now proves that endometriosis is a real disease with an array of physical symptoms. It's estimated that nearly 5.5 million women in the United States and Canada suffer from this disease.

Endometriosis occurs when abnormal growths of endometrial tissue (which normally lines the inside of the uterus) migrate outside of the uterus into the pelvic cavity. These growths are usually small and noncancerous, but in some women, they can cause extreme menstrual pain and other health problems, including infertility. The reason these growths are so troublesome is because they react to hormones just like normal uterine lining does. Like the uterine lining, these growths "shed" during menstruation, causing internal bleeding, inflammation and scarring. Endometrial growths can also spread to new areas, which explains why endometriosis is a progressive and chronic condition.

The cause of endometriosis is still a mystery, but theories include exposure to environmental estrogens like organochemicals. It may also include something called "retrograde menstruation" where menstrual tissue supposedly backs up into the fallopian tubes. While there are various theories behind its origin, we do know that endometriosis runs in families.

One of the most telling symptoms of endometriosis is pain *before* and during menstrual periods (worse than normal menstrual cramps), but other symptoms include:

• pain during sexual intercourse
• lower back pain with periods
• abdominal bloating and intestinal upset with periods
• pain during urination or bowel movements with periods
• pelvic tenderness
• abnormally heavy or irregular menstrual periods
• infertility

Endometriosis is the third leading cause of gynecologic hospitalization and often leads to a hysterectomy. Although treatments have varied over the years, doctors usually prescribe medications that lower estrogen and progesterone levels (e.g., birth control pills, anti-estrogens [Danazol], progestins and gonadotropin-releasing hormone [Leuprolide, Nafarelin]). Surgical treatments to remove endometrial growths, the ovaries or uterus may be necessary if symptoms are severe.

## My Endometriosis Treatment Strategy

If you suspect that you have endometriosis, ask your gynecologist to perform a laparoscopy to confirm the diagnosis. This is same-day surgery and only requires a tiny naval incision. Keep in mind that other diseases, including ovarian cancer, have symptoms similar to endometriosis. If the diagnosis is confirmed, consult with a gynecologist that specializes in treating the disease. Although conventional treatments for endometriosis may be necessary, depending on your situation, I always recommend starting with less invasive strategies for treatment.

Many of my patients have successfully dealt with the disease by changing their diet and beginning an exercise routine. Preliminary studies suggest that women who exercise two to four hours per week have a lower risk of developing endometriosis. I also advise women to cut out red meat, sugar and dairy foods, while including regular servings of coldwater fish, which contains fatty acids that act as natural anti-prostaglandin compounds. Remember that prostaglandins are the culprit chemicals that contribute to menstrual cramping.

Women with endometriosis should also use a strong natural progesterone cream. Ask your doctor for a prescription cream that can be custom-mixed by a pharmacist. Regular consumption of soy foods or supplementation with genistein is also essential. If you do

## The Anovulatory Cycle

□ ■ ■ ■

Too many healthy young women don't ovulate. Explanations range from the effect of xenoestrogens (environmental estrogens) to poor diets and chronic stress. I think it's a combination of all three. The major risk of anovulatory cycles (besides the fact that you can't conceive) is that it creates estrogen dominance, which can overstimulate the uterus and cause the formation of fibroids and abnormal uterine bleeding. If the problem isn't addressed promptly, your bones are also at risk. Failing to ovulate at a young age is nothing to sneeze at. If the problem isn't addressed, you are putting yourself at risk for a variety of problems, including osteoporosis. Moreover, you need to find out if any ovarian disease is present, and the sooner the better.

decide to try surgical treatments, consider having a laparoscopy, which involves cutting out the abnormal tissue or destroying it with a laser, before even thinking about a hysterectomy.

## Infertility Issues

One of the most difficult things a woman can face is the inability to conceive. She may face years of unsuccessful and costly treatments, constant emotional highs and lows, and insensitivity on the part of family and friends. And its causes are diverse—hormone abnormalities, low thyroid function, endometriosis, scarring of the fallopian tubes, to name a few. Low sperm counts or the complete absence of sperm in men also account for more than 35 percent of infertility problems.

Unfortunately, infertility rates are rising. I was surprised to learn that one in thirteen couples is infertile. Infertility is technically defined as the failure to become pregnant after a year of unprotected intercourse. If you have been trying to get pregnant for at least a year and have been unsuccessful, speak with a doctor. If you decide to try an infertility treatment program, first schedule a test to ensure your fallopian tubes aren't blocked. If they are, all the fertility drugs in the world won't do a thing. At the same time, request a hormone profile (a simple blood test) to see if a hormone imbalance is at the heart of the problem. If you continually skip your periods and have excessive facial hair, you may be producing too much testosterone. Additionally, check your iron levels. Low iron has been linked to infertility. Finally, be sure to also have your husband's sperm count checked.

## Traditional Treatments for Infertility

Conventional treatment options for infertility include using fertility drugs such as clomiphene (Clomid, Serophene), gonadorelin (Factrel, Lutrepulse), human chorionic gonadotropin or "hCG" (APL, Fullutein, Humegon, Pregnyl, Profasi), and human menopausal gonadotropins or "hMG" (Metrodin, Pergonal, and Repronal). Doctors may also recommend artificial insemination, which involves placing sperm through the cervix into the uterus. In a more complex and expensive procedure called "in vitro fertilization," the egg is collected from the ovary and fertilized in a petri dish. The fertilized embryo is then implanted into the uterus.

These treatments have enabled many women to conceive and represent one of medicine's most miraculous advances. Unfortunately, many of these treatments are costly and are rarely covered by insurance. Infertility treatments typically involve repeated pelvic exams, inseminations, sustained hormone treatments and in some cases, multiple surgeries. Yes, these treatments are challenging, but they pale in comparison to the emotional component of the experience. Women tell me all the time that trying to get pregnant was the most emotionally draining experience of their lives. When a woman is faced with the prospect that she may never have a child, she can become severely depressed. And her attempts to become pregnant can eclipse everything else in her life, putting an enormous strain on her marriage. "I became totally obsessed with getting pregnant" one of my patients told me. "My life became a roller coaster ride of high hopes followed by deep disappointment." While I wholeheartedly support conventional treatments for infertility, I like to see women improve their odds for conception by making a few crucial lifestyle changes.

## Eating to Get Pregnant

Women who are trying to get pregnant should make a conscious effort to eat more fruits and vegetables. They should also include more plant sources of protein, like legumes (i.e. soybeans, lentils, split peas and the like). And get off the caffeine! New studies reveal that drinking less than two cups of coffee a day can result in delayed conception. Caffeine has also been linked to endometriosis. Another study found that women who consumed more than one cup of coffee per day had a 50 percent reduction in fertility.

Alcohol is also problematic. Moderate consumption of alcohol may be acceptable, but if you're having trouble conceiving, don't drink at all. One study found that women who consumed alcohol had more than a 50-percent drop in the probability of conception than those who did not.

# Kick the Habit

If you smoke, stop. Simply stated, the more you smoke, the less likely you are to get pregnant. And your chances are even worse if your mother smoked. Research shows that women whose mothers smoked during their pregnancy are less likely to conceive compared with those whose mothers were nonsmokers. Moreover, if you do get pregnant, you can't smoke anyway, so why wait?

# Consider Natural Compounds

According to a double-blind study, women taking a multivitamin-mineral supplement increase their fertility rate. You should also consider the possibility that you suffer from deficiencies of certain key vitamins and minerals necessary for conception. For example, a vitamin E deficiency can cause infertility. In fact, one trial in which infertile couples were given vitamin E (200 IU per day for the female and 100 IU per day for the male) reported a significant increase in conception. As I mentioned before, low iron levels may also interfere with fertility.

While more studies are needed, the data on PABA (para-aminobenzoic acid) supplementation (at 100 mg four times per day) is compelling. Supplementing with PABA may increase the ability of estrogen to facilitate fertility. And if you're going to be doing artificial insemination or in vitro, supplementation with the amino acid L-arginine may improve your chances of fertilization. Of course, consult with your doctor before beginning a supplement program. And be sure to check for side effects or other interactions, especially if you are currently undergoing conventional infertility treatments.

Chapter 11

□ ▨ ▪ ▪

# Cancer and Women: Improving the Odds

In the community of living tissues, the uncontrolled mob of misfits
that is cancer behaves like a gang of perpetually wilding adolescents.
They are the juvenile delinquents of cellular society.
– *Sherwin B. Nuland*

**Maggie was sixty-two** years old when she first came to me. It didn't take long to figure out that she had ovarian cancer. Like most women facing the prospect of cancer, Maggie was terrified. The truth is, ovarian cancer is a scary prospect—the majority of patients live less than three years after diagnosis. But unlike most patients, who typically are offered the option of one or a combination of therapies—surgery, chemotherapy and radiation therapy—I encouraged Maggie to also take a nutritional supplement called transfer factor in addition to her chemotherapy. (See Chapter 16 for more info on transfer factor.)

To make a long story short, Maggie has done remarkably well. Moreover she has continued to take transfer factor to this day (and it's the only thing she takes—no other drugs or supplements). It's eight years later, and Maggie is still cancer free! Over the course of my practice, I can count on one hand the number of women who've had ovarian cancer and survived past two years. The addition of transfer factor fortified Maggie's immune system, improving her response to chemo and radiation and bettering her ability to fight off a recurrence of her cancer.

While Maggie's story may seem too good to be true, the fact is I've seen similar results in other patients who use transfer factor and other "complementary" therapies while undergoing conventional treatments. I'm not saying that transfer factor or any other supplement can cure cancer, but numerous studies conclusively show that it can make a difference. Why do I recommend such therapies for something as serious as cancer? Well, for the very reason that cancer is serious. For many women, it's a life-or-death scenario. They know their odds, so they're willing to try something—even if the FDA won't look at it—that has a credible track record.

Informing a woman that she will most likely die of cancer is a very sobering experience. While delivering a cancer diagnosis is bad enough, I also feel a great deal of frustration because undoubtedly, many of these cases could have been prevented, more effectively treated, or their recurrence prevented with complementary therapies like diet modification and specific nutritional supplements. I firmly believe that a physician not only bears the responsibility of sharing all treatment options with a cancer patient, they also have a moral obligation to inform all women how they can reduce their risk of cancer and cancer recurrence. I call it protection through prevention.

Before we discuss my recommendations for both preventing and treating cancer, let's take a quick look at female-specific cancers.

## A Breast Cancer Epidemic

Breast cancer is one of the most serious health threats facing North American women today. While we do have an earlier diagnosis and slightly higher cure rate, the number of new cases of breast cancer continues to increase every year. Over 200,000 women were diagnosed with breast cancer in 2002 versus 198,000 in 2001. And regarding cancer deaths in women, breast cancer is currently second only to lung cancer.

After years of research, scientists concede that only 25 percent of breast cancer cases can be traced to a specific cause. Heredity accounts for approximately 5 percent of all cases. If breast cancer runs in your immediate family, your risk is certainly higher. What you eat, whether you smoke, and when you started and ended your periods are also factored in the risk equation. Moreover, exposure to certain levels of radiation can make you more vulnerable. But even when one takes all of these factors into account, the vast majority of breast cancer cases continue to baffle doctors. This is why I believe that it's most wise to fight breast cancer before it strikes.

## Breast Cancer: Predetermined or Not?

"It's in my genes" seems to be the popular way to explain how and why we get cancer. But don't assume that if cancer runs in your family, your fate is set in stone. It is now believed that genetic programming does not necessarily imply genetic determination. Dr. Jeffrey Bland, a leading clinical nutritionist, said "We are given a genetic map, but within that map there are many different routes." What Dr. Bland is telling us is that our health destiny depends on the lifestyle and dietary choices we make—not solely on our genetic signature.

The fact is that our general genetic make-up has not changed significantly over the last 200 years, yet we are seeing a tremendous increase in the incidence of breast cancer. Okay. Let's assume that you've inherited the "breast cancer gene." What next? While you may be predisposed to the disease, keep in mind that certain factors can trigger or aggravate genetic abnormalities. In other words, exposure to certain hormones, chemicals and what you choose to eat or not eat can disrupt normal cell division and stimulate the growth of cancer.

Rather than taking drugs or having surgery, the less heroic measures of altering diet, lifestyle and environmental factors may well prove to be more useful. Donald C. Malins, director of molecular epidemiology at the Pacific Northwest Research Foundation in Seattle, blames most breast cancer on free-radical damage to breast cell DNA. He believes this damage is likely to be what turns the BRCA1 and BRCA2 genes bad as well (these genes normally suppress breast and ovarian cancer). He also believes that diets rich in antioxidants neutralize free radicals and could be very helpful during early stages of DNA damage. Using more powerful and concentrated antioxidants when the damage is more advanced may also help repair DNA damage.

I believe that women with a genetic tendency for breast cancer are more susceptible to environmental triggers than "normal" women. Remove the triggers, however, and their inherited tendency has less opportunity to express itself.

## A Smoking Gun

Recent research shows that long-term smokers (who smoke twenty cigarettes a day) have four times the risk of developing breast cancer if they have a particular mutation of the NAT2 gene, which impairs their ability to neutralize carcinogens. About 50 percent of Caucasian women, 35 percent of black women, 20 percent of Chinese women, and 10 percent of Asian women have this gene mutation. The massive upswing in the number of teenage girls who smoke will most certainly impact breast cancer cases. Keep in mind that it is the breast tissue of younger women that is most sensitive to carcinogens.

So, back to the idea that there is much a woman can do to con-

## Breast Tissue is Vulnerable

□ ▪ ■ ■

Breast tissue is very sensitive and thus vulnerable to the effects of many outside factors. One of these is radiation damage, and the experience following the atomic bombs at Hiroshima and Nagasaki illustrates this vulnerability—a very high proportion of female survivors later developed breast cancer. Questions are also being raised regarding EMFs (electromagnetic fields) created by everyday items like computers, fax machines, and mobile phones and their impact on breast cancer. There is enough concern for the World Health Organization to have set up a five-year study examining all the health issues relating to EMFs.

Xenoestrogens—synthetic compounds that behave similarly to estrogen—may also contribute to cancer. These substances come from chemical sources like petrochemical products and readily accumulate in the fatty tissue of the breast. There, they mimic estrogen by stimulating the replication of mutated cells. For this reason alone, consistently supplementing with an estrogen blocker is crucial. Phytoestrogens like those found in soy provide this kind of protection. They attach to receptor cells found in the breast, thereby not allowing the dangerous xenoestrogens to do the same. Common xenoestrogens include:

- fat soluble hormones in meat
- DDT
- PCBs (polychlorinated biphenyls)
- cosmetics
- foaming agents in soap and detergents
- plastic cookware
- various pesticides and herbicides
- birth control pills
- condom spermicides

trol how her genes express—or behave—themselves. Doctors need to tell their patients that lifestyle choices, eating habits, and exercise can all positively influence gene expression. While we can do nothing about choosing our genetic background, we can do everything about changing our "genetic fate."

## Breast Cancer Risk Factors

- early onset of periods
- late pregnancy
- no pregnancies
- obesity
- use of hormone replacement therapy
- late menopause
- radiation exposure
- long-term use of oral contraceptives
- high exposure to toxins
- family history/genetic disposition
- lack or dysfunction of a tumor-suppressing gene
- the presence of BRCA1 and BRCA2 gene mutations

## Conventional Treatments for Breast Cancer

Women with noninvasive breast cancer, also known as *ductal carcinoma in situ,* are typically treated with surgery. Chemotherapy and radiation are added for more extensive cases. A breast cancer treatment strategy hinges on how invasive or potentially fatal the cancer is. Treatment philosophies are constantly in flux, so what was considered standard protocol yesterday may be thought of as obsolete today.

## A Breaking News Announcement

□ ▨ ■ ■

As I was writing this chapter, scientists at the University of Washington announced that a whopping 60 percent of women with breast cancer are missing something called a "tumor suppressing gene." In other words, they are missing the genetic material that keeps a breast tumor from growing. The good news is that through the progress of genetic medicine, adding that gene back to the body may be possible. The real question is why that tumor suppressing gene is missing or malfunctioning in the first place.

Remember this—anything that increases breast tissue turnover (principally estrogens and xenoestrogens) also increases your risk of developing breast cancer. We must also consider the notion that external estrogens coupled with bad food choices may be impairing the function of tumor suppressing genes. Moreover, remember that a free radical will grab an electron from anywhere it can find one. Perhaps its target is a tumor-suppressing cell. Consequently the cell's structure could become damaged and its protective actions compromised.

## Forms of Mastectomy

The term "mastectomy" simply refers to the surgical removal of the breast or breast tissue and affected axillary (under arm) lymph nodes. In some cases, women who have had a breast removed are also advised to undergo chemotherapy and radiation treatments. There are four types of mastectomies—simple, modified radical, radical and lumpectomy.

## Simple Mastectomy

This surgery involves the removal of the breast tissue, skin and nipple. The lymph nodes are usually not affected. Frequently this type of mastectomy is done to prevent breast cancer in a woman with a very high risk. A woman who's had a simple mastectomy may opt for breast reconstruction or she may be fitted for a breast prosthesis.

## Modified Radical Mastectomy

This is the most common type of mastectomy and involves the complete removal of the breast, nipple and areola and varying amounts of lymph node tissue under the arm. The size of the incision can vary from one to eight inches in length. Modified radical mastectomies are performed when conserving breast tissue is not an option.

## Radical Mastectomy

This is the most invasive mastectomy and involves the removal of the breast tissue, skin, nipple, areola, lymph nodes and underlying chest muscle. Decades ago, this was the most common surgical approach to treat breast cancer. Today, we know that it is rarely necessary and should only be used in cases of advanced breast disease. Interestingly, survival rates of this type of mastectomy compared to less radical ones appears to be the same.

## Lumpectomy or Partial Mastectomy (also known as breast conserving surgery)

A partial mastectomy (more commonly known as a *lumpectomy*) involves the removal of only the breast tissue that contains the lump and some lymph nodes. While the surgery may be effective, it can also leave poor cosmetic results if the tumor is large in relation to the size of the breast. Just as a side note, a recent long-term study found that there appears to be little or no difference in survival rates between women who have a lumpectomy and those who have a mastectomy. I strongly suggest discussing these findings with your doctor.

## Factors that Determine Type of Breast Cancer Surgery

• stage of cancer
• lymph node involvement
• tumor size
• type of tumor
• histological grade of the tumor
• whether the tumor is driven by estrogen or progesterone
• prior treatment with radiation
• overall health

## Chemotherapy

Chemotherapy is typically used for all breast cancer patients, regardless of the disease stage, and is almost always administered after surgery. Simply stated, chemo is the use of chemicals, or drugs, that destroy cancer cells. These drugs work by preventing cancer cells from growing or multiplying. Their major drawback is that they can't distinguish diseased cells from healthy ones. The inevitable destruction of healthy cells contributes to side effects like nausea, baldness, and extreme fatigue.

Frequently, two or more chemo drugs are administered simultaneously to achieve maximal effect. Your cancer is considered cured if you remain free of any evidence of cancer cells after

## The Protein Promise

□ ▪ ■ ■

There is potentially good news in the area of cancer diagnosis. Researchers have determined that many women with breast or ovarian cancer have an abnormal protein profile. In fact, those women with early stages of the diseases have a very similar or identical profile. This suggests that soon we'll be able to predict who will get cancer before the disease actually develops. I recently spoke with a researcher from an Ivy League school who believes that within five years, protein profiling will be available to high-risk individuals and will eventually become part of routine screening tests.

The only negative aspect of this remarkable diagnostic tool is making the difficult decision of what to do if you test positive for the protein profile but have no signs of cancer. Do you opt for something as radical as a mastectomy even though you don't have cancer? Certainly, knowing that cancer looms on your horizon would prompt vigorous preventive measures. Interestingly, abnormal protein profiles have also been linked to Alzheimer's and prostate disease. It wouldn't surprise me if free radical damage also contributed to the formation of these abnormal proteins—a probability that further supports the use of diet and specific supplements, especially antioxidants, to prevent cancer.

treatment. While chemo is usually recommended after breast surgery, it can be used alone or with radiation treatments. It may also be employed to shrink a tumor prior to surgery. Chemotherapy drugs include combinations of doxorubicin (Adriamycin, Rubex, Doxil), cyclophosphamide (Cytoxan, Neosar), methotrexate (Folex, Rheumatrex), and fluorouracil (5-FU, Adrucil, Efudex, Fluoroplex).

# Talking About Tamoxifen

Tamoxifen (Nolvadex) is also recommended for long-term use in women whose cancer is estrogen driven. Tamoxifen is taken in pill form and interferes with the production of estrogen and interferes with the binding of estrogen to breast cells. After breast surgery and chemotherapy, it is commonly prescribed for a number of years. Tamoxifen is generally considered effective but comes with considerable side effects—increased risk of uterine cancer, phlebitis, cataracts, and bone weakness. If you choose to go on tamoxifen therapy, I would suggest adding genistein. While some might question this recommendation, I believe that the preferential binding of genistein to estrogen receptors can enhance tamoxifen's desired effect while lessening its side effects. I currently have four patients on tamoxifen, and I tell them to use genistein as a safeguard. While tamoxifen decreases estrogen stimulation in breast tissue, it appears to do just the opposite in the uterine lining. Genistein, on the other hand, helps discourage an overgrowth of the uterine lining, thereby decreasing a woman's risk of endometrial cancer—a risk factor when taking tamoxifen.

Ironically, even hormone-inhibiting drugs designed to prevent breast cancer may stimulate cancer growth elsewhere. In his book, *The Breast Cancer Prevention Diet,* Dr. Bob Arnot points out that while potent estrogen-blocking drugs like tamoxifen can help prevent breast cancer, it can double the rate of uterine cancer in some women.

In more advanced cases of breast cancer, other drugs that block the production of estrogen may also be used and include exemestane (Aromasin), vorazole (Rizivor), letrozole (Femara), anastrozole (Arimidex), and formestane (Lentaron).

## Tamoxifen, Birth Control Pills and Cancer

As a gynecologic oncologist, I have seen a frightening increase in breast cancer occurrence. I have no doubt that synthetic estrogen exposure (both from environmental and pharmaceutical sources) is directly involved in this. In fact, I'm currently treating five women who were on prescription hormone therapies when they developed cancer—something that's not supposed to happen.

If you took older generation birth-control pills, you may also have an increased breast cancer risk if the disease runs in your family. In one study of 426 families, researchers found that oral contraceptive use tripled breast cancer risk among women with sisters or mothers who had the disease. This increased suscepti-bility usually applies to women who used birth control pills before the early seventies. Today's oral contraceptives have lower doses of estrogen and progestin, although their long-term safety is still in question. After all is said and done, I believe that the sin-gle most important factor linked to breast cancer is the exposure of breast tissue to estrogen. Consequently, I'm continually get-ting on my soap box to preach the value of natural estrogen blockers like isoflavones.

# Mammograms: Detection, Not Prevention

When it comes to mammograms, I believe we have a mixed bag. For instance, 20 percent of breast cancer cases don't show up on mammogram screenings. In addition, there is considerable controversy as to when to start having them. The American Medical Association recommends annual mammograms for all women age forty and older. Some experts argue that forty is too young. Why? Because the breast tissue of a pre-menopausal woman is more dense and less fatty than that of postmenopausal women, and thus can more easily hide or camouflage a tumor.

This makes reading a mammogram more prone to errors—either false positives or missed positives can result. The truth is that less than 5 percent of women under age fifty whose mammograms come back abnormal actually have breast cancer. For women over fifty, the statistic is 15 percent higher.

The real question is, "Do mammograms save lives?" Sure they do, but the numbers aren't that impressive, especially when it comes to premenopausal women. If breast cancer runs in your family, you'll want annual screenings. And there is new technology that can improve our abilities to detect cancer. Keep in mind that emerging diagnostic techniques, including milk duct aspirations as well as examination of ducts with tiny telescopes, may provide better detection than mammograms. To make things more complicated, much controversy looms over the safety of mammograms, which expose breast tissue to low-level radiation.

Personally, I believe mammograms can be a life-saver. But they are somewhere in-between the "after-the-fact" mentality and a true preventive approach. Here's my pitch—instead of aggressively pushing for annual mammograms, why don't we put just as much emphasis on prevention? We should teach our girls to eat healthy—avoid saturated fats, emphasize phytoestrogenic foods like soy, and increase intake of raw fruits and vegetables (especially those high in lycopene and carotene like tomatoes and carrots and cruciferous vegetables like cabbage, cauliflower and broccoli). We should encourage them to not smoke and to avoid alcohol. And we should educate them about the many health benefits of regular exercise. If we did, breast cancer rates would dramatically decline. It's that simple.

## Overlooking Ovarian Cancer

Ovarian cancer is one of the deadliest cancers that strike women. This is so primarily because the cancer develops undetected until it's too late. A recent study of nearly 2,000 women with ovarian cancer revealed that they had a complete set of symptoms—abdominal bloating, pain and abnormal bleeding— long before they were properly diagnosed with the disease.

Keep in mind that if ovarian cancer is caught early enough, survival rates can be as high as 90 percent. Unfortunately, only one fourth of women with ovarian cancer find out before the disease has spread beyond the ovaries, something that severely reduces their chances of survival. That's why it's so important to have any abnormal symptoms checked out. And insist that your doctor considers all possibilities. Sadly, doctors fail to detect ovarian cancer in about 80 percent of women during their first visit. The rest are simply misdiagnosed.

Unfortunately, there is no good way to detect ovarian cancer in its early stages. A blood test, called CA125, may be helpful but currently it's not economically feasible. Pelvic exams and ultrasounds are the best way to discover the disease.

## What's My Risk of Ovarian Cancer?

About one in fifty-seven North American women will develop ovarian cancer. Most of them will be over the age of fifty, but younger women can develop the disease. There are a number of things that raise your risk of ovarian cancer. They include:

• age (your risk increases with your age)
• postmenopausal hormone therapy (especially estrogen alone)
• fertility drugs
• family history of ovarian cancer (higher risk if mother or sister has had ovarian cancer; somewhat higher if other relatives, such as grandmother, developed the disease)
• personal history of colorectal cancer
• lack of pregnancies and/or breastfeeding

## The Role of Heredity in Breast and Ovarian Cancer

□ ▪ ▪ ▪

Within the last decade, scientists have discovered gene mutations that appear in families prone to breast and ovarian cancer. Earlier in the chapter, we discuss some of these genes—called BRCA1 and BRCA2—and their mutations. If a woman has a BRCA1 mutation, this means her overall risk of breast cancer is 56–78 percent and 16–60 percent for ovarian cancer. Keep in mind, however, that only 2–3 percent of women with breast cancer have BRCA mutations, so other factors are obviously at play. What action you take if your have a BRCA1 or BRCA2 mutation is highly debatable, although having a mastectomy will reduce your breast cancer risk by 90 percent. Likewise, if you have the gene mutation, removing the ovaries is probably a good idea. As mentioned earlier, a missing tumor suppressing gene may also explain why breast cancer runs in some families.

# Ovarian Cancer and Vegetable Consumption

As you know by now, I firmly believe that educating our public as to the advantages of disease prevention, especially from a young age, can produce tremendous benefits. For instance, one study shows that women who consume at least two and a half servings of fruit and vegetables daily as adolescents are 46 percent less likely to develop ovarian cancer. Why aren't we getting the word out? Can you imagine the market for a drug that could prevent disease that well? The study also suggests that dangerous free radicals are at work early in a girl's life, so eating the right foods at the right time is crucial. Considering how most teenage girls today eat (or don't eat), their future health prospects aren't too bright.

Another study singles out carotenes and lycopene (found in foods like carrots and tomatoes) and their potential role in preventing ovarian cancer, especially in postmenopausal women. Not surprisingly, carotenes and lycopene are powerful antioxidants. An easy way to raise your lycopene intake is to eat more tomato products (especially tomato sauces), and carotenes are found in a number of foods, such as carrots, squash, cantaloupe, apricots, sweet potatoes, broccoli and many green leafy vegetables. I tell women to eat a minimum of five servings of carotene-rich vegetables and two half-cup servings of tomato sauce per week.

## Alecia's Story

Alecia came to see me from another state and had late-stage ovarian cancer. Women in her condition rarely live past two years. We removed the cancer surgically and then sent her for a course of chemo with transfer factor in one hand and genistein in the other. She sailed through the chemotherapy with minimal nausea and vomiting. More important is the fact that she has remained disease-free for three years, and her prognosis continues to look good.

## Buying More Time for Sarah

Three years ago, sixty-seven-year-old Sarah came to me with extensive, late-stage ovarian cancer. Due to a serious heart condition, surgery was out of the question, so I put her on minimal chemotherapy treatments combined with transfer factor and genistein. It's been three years now, and she's still alive. How much longer will she live? I don't know, but I really believe that, in light of how serious her cancer was, the transfer factor/genistein supplementation has bought her a significant amount of time.

# Cervical Cancer

Cervical cancer strikes over 14,000 women in this country every year. This type of cancer can be detected by having regular Pap smears, which reveal cell abnormalities signaling the development of the disease. Doctors use a variety of terms to describe abnormal cells found on the surface of the cervix. Squamous intraepithelial lesion (SIL) refers to an area of abnormal tissue where mutated cells are found only in the surface layer. Changes that occur in these cells are usually placed into two categories:

- Low-grade SIL: Refers to early changes in the size, shape, and number of cells that form the surface of the cervix. Many of these lesions will disappear with no treatment. Some, however, may grow and continue to change, forming what is called a high-grade lesion. Precancerous low-grade lesions are also called mild dysplasia or cervical intraepithelial neoplasia 1 (CIN 1). These early changes are primarily seen in women under thirty.

- High-grade SIL: This term refers to the presence of more advanced precancerous cells on the surface of the cervix. It usually takes years for these kinds of cells to become malignant and spread to deeper tissues of the cervix. High-grade lesions are also called moderate or severe dysplasia, CIN 2 or 3, or carcinoma in situ. They develop most often in women over the age of thirty.

When any abnormal cervical cells spread deeper into the cervix or other organs, the diagnosis is cervical cancer, or invasive cervical cancer, which occurs most often in women over the age of forty.

## Informed Consent?

■ ■ ■ ■

Cervical cancer is largely considered a sexually transmitted disease, and is usually passed via strains of the human papilloma virus. Since the sixties-spawned notion of free love, more and more young women are having sex at an earlier age. Consequently, their exposure to the virus that causes the disease is higher. Efforts are underway to develop vaccines for HPV but I believe that once again, prevention is better.

Meg Meeker, a pediatrician and author of a compelling book called *Epidemic: How Teen Sex is Killing Our Kids,* points out that sexually transmitted diseases among teens have become a full-blown epidemic and should be viewed as a nationwide emergency. She makes a strong case by citing some alarming numbers. In 1960, only two sexually transmitted diseases (STDs) were commonly seen in this country. Today, that number is thirty. If you care to know, one in five kids over the age of eleven has genital herpes—a 500 percent increase from 1976. Furthermore, after their first sexual encounter, studies reveal that teen-age girls have a 46 percent chance of contracting HPV.

As a physician, Dr. Meeker says that cervical abnormalities are routinely found in fifteen- and sixteen-year-old girls who've had multiple sexual partners. Consequently, she advocates teaching all girls that having sex in their teens puts them at higher risk for contracting HPV (not to mention a number of other STDs). Like her, I believe we should work to strongly discourage sexual promiscuity among teenagers.

# A Symptomless Disease

Unfortunately, symptoms of cervical cancer usually don't appear until the disease is in its later stages. Abnormal bleeding or vaginal discharge are the most common signs. For this reason, having a regular Pap smear and colposcopy (if the Pap results are abnormal) is a good idea. These procedures are painless and quick and should become an annual routine for all women who are sexually active, regardless of their age.

# What's My Risk of Cervical Cancer?

There are a number of things that can increase your risk of cervical cancer. They include the following:

- presence of human papilloma virus (HPV)
- multiple sexual partners
- long-term use of the pill
- smoking (doubles your risk)
- first time sexual intercourse at an early age
- poor socio-economic status
- multiple pregnancies
- pregnancy(ies) early in life

# Cervical Cancer—The Immune Connection

To cure or prevent any cancer, we must know what caused it in the first place. A virus called human papilloma virus, or HPV, appears to initiate cancer of the cervix. However, many women who have this virus never end up with cervical cancer. Why? Most likely because their diet and lifestyle all contribute to an optimally functioning immune system. Therefore, their defense

## Influencing Young People One at a Time

□ ▨ ▩ ▩

I believe we should work to strongly discourage sexual promiscuity among teenagers. Better yet, we should teach our children to remain celibate until they get married (yes, it is possible). And it's not just the negative physical impact that early sexuality can create—young people usually suffer significant emotional problems as well.

Doctors can play a key role in disease prevention by discussing the health risks of early sex with young women. Remember, the earlier a woman begins having sex, and the more sexual partners a woman has, the higher her risk of contracting the virus. A young woman is entitled to all the facts before she makes sexual decisions. In our politically-correct world, however, doctors often neglect to discuss "taboo" subjects with their patients.

Of course, parents can exert a tremendous influence on their children as well. A recent study showed that mothers can have a very positive influence in the sexual behavior of their children (especially their daughters.) My own daughter has become a quasi-vegetarian due to the example and belief system of my wife and me. (In fact, she asked me to come to her high school and give a talk to the kids on the merits of eating "vegetarian.") It truly is possible to influence the groundwork of how our children choose to conduct their lives.

systems are able to keep the virus in check. By contrast, women with HIV that contract HPV will often develop cervical cancer. In addition, women who smoke have a two-fold increase in their risk of getting cervical cancer. And we know that smoking can wreak havoc on the body's immune function. So, how do you prevent cervical cancer? Obviously, keeping your immune defenses in tip-top shape is crucial. In addition, quit smoking, eat more whole foods, exercise more, have regular Pap smears, take antioxidant supplements, and have "responsible" sex.

---

### Babies Having Babies

I'll never forget a consultation I had with Kelly and her mother. Kelly was fourteen years old and pregnant. She had been sexually active since she was eleven. Her mother was twenty-nine (you do the math). I did my darndest to convince Kelly that she should re-think her sexual decisions and delay having anymore sex. I gave her a graphic account of the many diseases she could contract and managed to get her attention. I figure that I probably succeeded in delaying Kelly's future sexual activity for about two years—not ideal, but better than nothing.

# Cervical Cancer Detection Made Easy

Years ago, I was approached by a small company that had developed a blood test for the detection of cervical cancer. Initially, I was skeptical, but decided anyway to verify their claim by using the test in my clinic. To my surprise, the test truly worked. It was designed to detect antibodies that had formed in response to the presence of HPV. In China, where cervical cancer is more prevalent than in the United States, more research on this blood test is underway and preliminary results are very encouraging. Additionally, research is underway at the University of Southern California School of Medicine and the Lahey Clinic in Massachusetts to confirm the exciting results from the Chinese studies.

The development of a sophisticated computer chip that can detect a number of sexually related diseases, including HIV, chlamydia, herpes, and HPV, through DNA channels is also in the works. These advances hopefully will make cervical cancer detection better and faster.

## Sometimes When You Win, You Lose

If every physician fully informed his or her patients of the dangers of having unprotected sex, the incidence of disease would surely decrease. To make my point—a physician friend of mine was given the assignment during WWII to work with soldiers at an army base in an effort to reduce the incidence of sexually-transmitted disease. His method? To show the soldiers graphic photos of the infection, tissue damage, and scarring caused by these diseases. The result? Sexually-transmitted disease rates on this base dropped to *zero*. Unfortunately, the commander of the base put a stop to my friend's program, not because it wasn't effective, but because he thought it was hurting recruiting campaigns. Within months, disease rates once again began to climb noticeably. The convoluted logic behind this decision still pervades our society today. Consequently, in our attempt to facilitate free choice, we have sacrificed a full disclosure of the truth.

## Calling an Audible for Janice

Back in my Sacramento days in the early 80's, I encountered Janice, who was fifty-five when we discovered that she had inoperable cervical cancer. The cancer had spread to her pelvic bone and could not be removed. It was one of those situations we referred to as a "peek and shriek" surgery. Put another way, when you see the extent of the cancer, you know there is little that can be done. We decided to take out all of Janice's reproductive organs, and then for the first time, we administered intra-operative radiation to the cancer that had invaded her pelvic bone. We had to think outside the box for this one—in other words, we threw out the playbook. While she was still under anesthesia, we wheeled her 500 feet to a "betatron" where, with the help of special devices, we directed high dose radiation straight at the cancer for two minutes. We had to stay clear of the room and placed her on a respirator (which we carefully monitored from a distance). After the radiation was delivered, we finished the operation in the treatment room. It was unconventional, to say the least. Happily, this combination of surgery and on-the-spot radiation completely cured her. When I last saw Janice (seven years after the surgery) she was still completely cancer-free.

## Uterine Cancer

Cancer of the uterus or endometrium occurs mostly in women over age fifty. Approximately 37,000 American women receive a diagnosis of uterine cancer each year, making it the fourth most common cancer found in women.

There are several risk factors for uterine cancer, but I believe the most significant by far is exposure to estrogen. That's why uterine cancer usually develops after a lifetime of estrogen exposure.

Abnormal vaginal bleeding is the most common symptom of uterine cancer. The discharge can start as a watery, blood-streaked flow that gradually contains more blood. Anytime you experience this type of postmenopausal bleeding, you should see your doctor. A biopsy of the endometrium may be needed, especially if the lining appears too thick.

As is the case with breast cancer, researchers have identified a gene variation that appears to nearly double a woman's risk of developing uterine cancer. Moreover, if you're overweight and carry this gene, you may be almost five times more likely to develop this type of cancer than leaner women. Fortunately, uterine cancer has one of the highest cure rates of all female cancers. Once again eating right, exercising and using a regimen of supplements like genistein and natural progesterone can help reduce your risk of this disease.

# What's My Risk of Uterine Cancer?

There are various types of uterine cancer, the most common being endometrial cancer, which begins in the lining of the uterus. All uterine cancers generally share the same risk factors. They include:

• increase in age (usually occurs after age fifty)
• endometrial hyperplasia, the thickening of the uterine lining
• use of estrogen therapy without progesterone
• obesity
• use of tamoxifen
• caucasian background
• colorectal cancer, especially hereditary forms
• absence of pregnancies
• menstruation early in life
• late menopause
• genetic mutation

---

### Avoid Progestins

■ ■ ■ ■

Synthetic progesterone, usually referred to as "progestins," add nothing beneficial to a woman who has undergone a hysterectomy and oophorectomy (removal of the ovaries). The bottom line is that she shouldn't take them. The same is true for postmenopausal women. Progestins don't protect women against breast cancer as many are led to believe. In fact, they may increase your risk of the disease. Can you tell that I'm not enthusiastic about progestins? By contrast, natural progesterone (which is chemically identical to the progesterone found in the human body) is beneficial for women of all ages.

Be aware that traditional HRT (hormone replacement therapy) may also raise your risk. Interestingly, the incidence of uterine cancer is higher in women with diabetes or high blood pressure (conditions that frequently accompany obesity).

## Optimizing Chemotherapy and Radiation Treatments

Unquestionably, if you receive chemotherapy treatments for any type of cancer, you become vulnerable to infections and a myriad of side effects like nausea and extreme fatigue. The chemicals not only seek and destroy the cancer cells, they also assault your immune system by lowering your white blood cell count. Chemotherapy also attacks any cells that multiply rapidly; for instance, those found in hair, the digestive system, and bone marrow.

While it defies all reason, most physicians don't prepare the body for chemotherapy and don't repair if afterwards. They simply prescribe a course of cell, tissue and immunity destruction and leave it at that. This makes no sense to me. When it comes to chemotherapy, physicians trained to heal the human body instead routinely prescribe therapies that poison and kill living cells. While sometimes this may be necessary, my gripe is that they totally neglect the use of diet, supplements and other therapies that can strengthen and protect the body before, both during and after treatments.

In fact, some physicians are so misinformed that they discourage patients from taking antioxidants during chemotherapy. Make no mistake, chemotherapy creates a glut of dangerous free radicals. Why shouldn't antioxidants be recommended? I've seen its benefits with many of my own patients, so much that I consider it a crucial component of any cancer therapy. I don't believe that taking these compounds will interfere in any way with the action of the chemotherapy. It will, however, help protect healthy cells from additional damage and support immune function.

## Treating Cancer Patients: My Thoughts

Let me stress here that I don't believe that any natural therapy can cure cancer of any kind. Having said that, let me also emphatically state that the use of complementary alternative therapies can significantly build the immune system and can prolong life or prompt cancer remission. Specific natural compounds can also help a cancer patient better tolerate chemotherapy and radiation and improve the overall quality of their life.

I want to also add that my theory regarding chemotherapy and subsequent cancer testing goes something like this—respect the patient's wishes, no matter what. In other words, doctors usually push chemotherapy until a patient's blood work shows no sign of cancer. If a patient refuses chemotherapy, why keep testing her blood? On several occasions, I've told women with cancer that if they stopped chemotherapy, they would die. Some have answered with "I don't give a damn, I'm done with this."

In these cases, it's vital to take the time to describe with complete honesty what the patient can expect as the disease progresses. Concerning the question, "How long do I have?" I inevitably reply, "I don't have the foggiest idea." A cancer patient who goes without treatment can last from two months to several years. The important thing is to support them in whatever course they choose to take.

Keep in mind that even a small nodule of cancer contains billions of cancer cells, and in order to kill just one cancer cell, the action of multiple immune cells is required. Optimizing our diets and taking a strong array of antioxidants, vitamins, minerals and immune-building supplements like transfer factor can make a world of difference in how a patient responds to chemotherapy.

---

## Gladys: Defying All Odds

Gladys was eighty-five and had extensive ovarian cancer. She couldn't really see the point of undergoing chemotherapy, and I empathized with her perspective. Because of her age and lack of transportation, I made a house-call from time to time to check up on her. As unorthodox as it sounds, I usually examined her on her living room couch. One day, I stopped by her home, and upon examining her I could find no sign of cancer. I was absolutely amazed, confounded and thrilled all at the same time. It appeared that without any treatment, the cancer had vanished—something I had never seen before.

# My Cancer Protocol

While I don't believe that any unconventional (or conventional, for that matter) therapy should be viewed as a cure for cancer, I know that specific therapies can make a dramatic difference in cancer prevention, treatment response, remission rates and overall health status. I want to reiterate that for most women, the three things that offer the greatest benefit in their fight against female-related cancers are to: (1) block estrogen receptors, (2) increase antioxidant intake, and (3) improve immune defenses. This can be done by using phytoestrogens like soy isoflavones (genistein), antioxidants like lycopene, and the immune booster transfer factor. I also strongly recommend optimizing your diet by making it high in vegetables, fruits, whole grains, coldwater fish, legumes and other "whole" foods.

I have seen time and time again that cancer patients who take these supplements and make these lifestyle changes do markedly better during chemotherapy and/or radiation treatments. If you have cancer and have decided to forgo conventional medicine altogether in exchange for natural treatments, keep in mind that

## The Townsend Family Cancer Chronicles

◻ ▪ ▪ ▪

Over the last forty years, I've treated thousands of women with various kinds of cancer. I've worked with them, designed their treatments and witnessed their improvement—or decline. I've shared in their joy when they won the fight and grieved when they lost it. My own life and those of several of my family members have all been profoundly touched by cancer. I lost my father and mother to cancer. I've had cancer and so has my son, my mother-in-law and sister-in-law. Experiencing the sting of a cancer diagnosis myself has allowed me to become a better, more compassionate caregiver for the women who seek my help when they become ill.

### There Are No Guarantees in Life

Trying to beat cancer is damn hard—not only for its victims but for anyone who loves them. Although my father was under the care of a team of top-notch doctors, ultimately, I was the one who decided which treatments he should pursue. This was no easy task. He was extremely well loved by his family and friends. In order to function in this capacity, I had to divorce my feelings—and so I put the walls up and kept my emotions in check. During his final weeks I felt tremendous pressure to find a way to somehow save his life. After all, I was a doctor.

I knew that my father had become gravely ill when he began doing strange things like eating soap. We soon discovered that the cancer had spread to his brain. Our options were limited. We could use a risky therapy that specifically targeted the brain tumors but could also kill him, or continue standard radiation treatments and hope for the best. The choice was mine alone. I decided on the high-risk treatment and prayed that it would work. It didn't and my father died from complications.

My mother also died of cancer and once again, I had to decide whether to fight her disease or let her die. Ten years ago on an October morning, she called and remarked that she could feel a lump in her breast. "Have you had a mammogram," I asked her. "No," she replied, "I was afraid that my Medicare wouldn't cover it." Tragically, her fears are echoed by scores of elderly women who avoid important medical tests for fear that they can't afford them. She did go in and the mammogram was positive. A simple lumpectomy cured her because the cancer was detected in its early stages. A decade later, a different kind of cancer would invade her body, and I would once again intervene in her behalf before her eventual death.

Several years ago, my mother-in-law found a lump in her breast. My wife and I took her to a radiologist where a biopsy was done and the diagnosis confirmed. The following day she had a mastectomy. Because her lymph nodes weren't affected, she didn't require any further treatments and made a full recovery. She eventually died from heart disease at the age of eighty-six.

Unfortunately, that would not be the end of our encounters with breast cancer. Four years ago, my wife's older sister Jan informed us that she had breast cancer. She also opted for a lumpectomy, followed by radiation therapy. Three years later, Jan developed a new malignancy in the same breast and had a mastectomy. While she was recovering, she died of a massive stroke.

Unfortunately Jan had been a long-time smoker, and ate poorly (her cholesterol level was over 400). She also took prescription drugs to control her hypertension, cholesterol, and pain. We made numerous attempts to get her to change her lifestyle, but she steadfastly refused and like so many other Americans, she paid the ultimate price. It's a well known fact that if a member of your immediate family develops cancer, your risk of cancer goes up. Joan's mother and sister had breast cancer and so

Joan's risk is considerable. For this reason, she has dramatically changed her diet and exercises more. In addition, she regularly takes genistein and natural progesterone.

### Do Unto Others

I believe in a special "golden rule" for physicians—choose the best possible course of treatment available for your patients and administer it with the same care and concern you'd show a member of your own family. That said, my own personal collective cancer experience with other doctors fell short of this mission statement. One of the most inhumane things a doctor can do is to put off calling a patient waiting for a possible cancer diagnosis.

### Call Me Tomorrow!

A few years ago, my son mentioned that his dermatologist had removed several moles from his back. As we conversed, his beeper went off and he was told to call his doctor. Instantly I knew that the moles were malignant. What made me furious was that his phone message told him to call after 24 hours. I was stunned at the insensitivity and total disregard shown by his physician. Making someone wait one minute longer than they have to for a potential life or death cancer diagnosis is reprehensible. Fortunately his melanoma was not advanced, so his chance of a cure was at least 98 percent. He had caught the melanoma early enough, but the moral of this story is that doctors should never, ever leave a phone message when the news is bad.

### The Shoe Was Now on the Other Foot

Before finding out if my suspicious mole was malignant or not, the sample was taken and I left town. When I received a message to call my office I knew why. I immediately phoned the pathologist and he confirmed my worst fears. I asked him how thick the melanoma was and he didn't know—he had sent my slides to a specialist in San Francisco. So I called the specialist's office and discovered that he was on vacation! I was now a patient who couldn't get in touch with his doctor. To say I was annoyed is an understatement. Due to my repeated calls, I was able to eventually contact him.

He thought my chance of recurrence was small—somewhere between 3 to 5 percent. I wasn't satisfied so I sent my slide to one of the world's premier experts on malignant melanoma. His conclusion—my cancer was much worse than I'd been told and my chances of survival were slim. Now I was in another dilemma frequently faced by patients—what do I believe? Not surprisingly, I went with the more optimistic consensus. Make no mistake, however, twelve years later I still wonder.

### Channeling the Fear Factor for Good

There isn't a day that goes by that I don't think about my cancer. Any time I discover a lump or bump, or feel aches or pains, I assume, "this is it." Only one patient out of thousands that I've treated for cancer says she doesn't worry about a recurrence, and I don't believe her. Am I scared that my cancer will return? You bet I am. Fear is a common denominator among cancer victims. I saw it on my wife's face when her mother was diagnosed. I saw it in my son when he got that dreaded phone call. And I've seen it on the face of every woman to whom I've had to break the bad news. The important thing is to transform your fear into a driving force that affects lifestyle changes that protect the body from cancer. Talk to your doctor, write letters to your insurance company, form a support group, get the word out and last but not least—don't be afraid to take charge of your own health.

## Why Don't We Have a Cure for Cancer?

Concerning cancer, a man named Auden said, "Nobody knows what the cause is, though some pretend they do; it is like some hidden assassin waiting to strike at you. Childless women get it, and men when they retire; it is as if there had to be some outlet for their foiled creative fire." By the year 2000, cancer is expected to kill one million Americans per year, overtaking heart disease as the leading cause of death.

We don't have a cure for cancer and probably won't get one for years. It all boils down to money. While genetic research and other avenues look promising, a real cancer cure is barely visible on the horizon and when it emerges, must be FDA approved and patented. You know where I stand on this. Currently the only way to make big money off of a remedy is to patent it. Dietary supplements are not "patentable" so big companies aren't interested in pursuing any of them as potential cancer cures. Consequently, vital studies that might show the cancer-curing potential of a natural compound are not funded by the big guys.

Over the last three decades, we've spent over $30 billion for a cancer cure, and I'm not sure we're any closer to it than when we started. When it comes to cancer research, I believe that we haven't been able to see the forest for the trees. Scores of studies tell us that environmental chemicals found in plastics, pesticides, foods, and water can negatively impact the endocrine system and contribute to hormone-driven cancers. Moreover, other pollutants can stimulate a variety of other malignancies in other body systems. Exposure to these chemicals coupled with poor eating choices makes for a lethal cocktail of carcinogens. So far, it's been a losing battle. Until we learn the basic biochemistry of the cell and how to protect that cell, cancer will always be with us, even in the post genome world.

if your tumors are advanced, you may not be able to effectively cope with the cancer—no matter how many supplements you take. For this reason, you might consider surgery to remove the cancer and then opt for an aggressive course of immune-building supplements, dietary changes, and other alternative approaches. My philosophy is to use the best of both worlds to fight cancer, but you must ultimately decide.

# Suggested Supplements for Cancer Patients

### Transfer Factor

This immune molecule, isolated from cow colostrum, adds data to the human immune system's memory banks. Improving immune function is critical when fighting cancer. John Bailar, M.D., Ph.D., and former editor-in-chief of the *Journal of the National Cancer Institute* has said, "For cancer to start and then continue growing, it must outmaneuver the many long arms of your immune defenses. The immune system is both your first and last defense against cancer." For anyone undergoing surgery, chemotherapy and/or radiation, transfer factor supplementation can make a real difference. Dozens of studies show that transfer factor can substantially improve immune function. Japanese and Chinese clinical studies have found that the immunosuppression that results from chemotherapy can be lessened by using transfer factor. Italian, Japanese and American studies demonstrate that the use of transfer factor to enhance immunity after cancer surgery significantly improves the chances of a cancer-free future. Take six to eight 200-mg capsules per day. (See Chapter 16 for more information on transfer factor.)

## Genistein and Daidzein (Soy Isoflavones)

I believe that genistein and daidzein are two of the most powerful weapons we have against estrogen-induced cancers. Both of these isoflavones inhibit the proliferation of breast cancer cells in scores of test tube studies. In addition, the overwhelming majority of animal studies report that soy isoflavones protect against mammary cancer in a variety of ways.

One of the best ways to fight or prevent cancer is to block the action of estrogen on hormone-sensitive tissue. Genistein is one of nature's most powerful estrogen blockers; therefore, it only stands to reason that it could discourage the growth of estrogen-driven female cancers. A 1997 study published in *Nutrition and Cancer* reported that while genistein has only one one-thousandth the hormonal potency of human estrogen, it can still attach to breast cell receptors thereby preventing their contact with the body's more dangerous estrogens (not to mention protection against exposure to environmental estrogens—called xenoestrogens—as well). Because soy isoflavones act as weak estrogens, some doctors discourage their use for women with cancer. I heartily disagree. Just look at Asian women who have survived breast cancer and never stopped eating soy. There is no evidence that consuming soy isoflavones contributed to the disease in these women.

In fact, I would propose that just the opposite is true when it comes to genistein and daidzein. Not only can genistein block the action of estrogen on breast tissue, it also sports an impressive array of other anticancer properties. Genistein prevents cancer cell growth by inhibiting the activity of tyrosine protein kinase and other enzymes involved in the formation of cancerous tumors. Moreover, research findings indicate that genistein slows down angiogenesis (the formation of new blood vessels that nourish a tumor), thereby causing the tumor to shrink. And last but not least, genistein possesses powerful antioxidant actions that protect cells from dangerous free radicals, which can stimulate the growth of cancer (and are created in large amounts during chemotherapy and radiation treatments). Genistein's sidekick, daidzein, also reduces the risk of cancer because it stimulates lymphocyte activity in a way that genistein alone can't—suggesting that the two compounds should be consumed together. Simply put, I believe that soy isoflavones offer a number of cancer-fighting actions for women. And when it comes to taking isoflavones to protect against cancer, the sooner the better. A study conducted at the Comprehensive Cancer Center in Birmingham, Alabama, and published in 1998, concluded that taking genistein during the early years (prepuberty) offered significant protection to laboratory animals from chemically induced cancer.

Because of the controversy surrounding the use of pharmaceutical estrogen-blockers like tamoxifen for women who have had breast cancer, soy isoflavones offer a very promising alternative. Clearly, women with breast cancer need to block estrogen. Consequently, I tell my patients to take a genistein/daidzein supplement. I have absolutely no doubt that phytoestrogenic isoflavones will play a major role in decreasing the incidence of hormone-stimulated cancers without the risks associated with estrogen-blocking drugs. Genistein and daidzein are available in capsulized form, and most products contain a combination of both.

## Natural Progesterone

A study published in the *American Journal of Epidemiology* conducted at Johns Hopkins Medical School in 1981 compared women with low progesterone to those that had normal levels. It found that the occurrence of breast cancer was nearly five and a half times higher in the women who lacked progesterone. The researchers concluded that the women low in progesterone had a ten-fold increase for *all* female cancers combined. Recent studies have also suggested that women who use estrogenic drugs double their risk of breast cancer. Even the addition of progestins does not appear to reduce that risk. By contrast, using natural progesterone has the opposite effect. It doesn't appear to alter hormone-sensitive tissue in a negative way. Without question, the protective action of natural progesterone is an absolute must for any woman who doesn't ovulate, has estrogen dominance, or needs hormone replacement.

Moreover, post-hysterectomy women also need to consider natural progesterone. Misguided physicians believe that progesterone replacement is not necessary for women who have had their uterus and ovaries removed—nothing could be further from the truth. These women are often placed on traditional HRT (hormone replacement therapy that contains progestins).

## Vitamin D

Breast cancer rates appear to be higher in areas where women are exposed to less sunlight. Sunlight is what stimulates the formation of vitamin D in the skin. In animal studies, vitamin D-like compounds have actually prevented the formation of breast cancer.

Topical vitamin D ointments may also protect breast tissue. In a preliminary trial, activated vitamin D was applied to the breasts of nineteen patients with breast cancer once daily for six weeks. Of the fourteen patients who completed the trial, three showed a substantial reduction in tumor size, and one showed a minor improvement. (If you're interested in this, you can get a prescription to have activated vitamin D included in a topical ointment.)

Vitamin D supplementation also enhances both the ability of tamoxifen to block estrogen and the effectiveness of chemotherapy treatments.

Take 1,000 IU daily.

## Coenzyme Q10 (CoQ10)

French researchers have reported that the lower a woman's blood level of coenzyme Q10, the higher her chances of a breast cancer recurrence. Studies of women with breast cancer suggest that coQ10 supplements (in addition to conventional treatment) may help shrink tumors and contribute to a partial remission. Scientists at the University of Texas in Austin conducted a study with thirty-two patients, aged thirty-two to eighty-one, whose breast cancer had spread to their lymph nodes. They were given an "adjuvant nutritional protocol" in addition to standard surgery and chemotherapy for eighteen months. The daily nutrients added to their treatment were 2,850 mg of vitamin C, 2,500 mg of vitamin E, 58 mg of beta-carotene, 387 mcg of selenium (plus secondary vitamins and minerals), 1.2 grams of gamma linolenic acid, 3.5 grams of omega-3 fatty acids, and 90 mg of coenzyme Q10. Six of the patients showed partial tumor regression. In addition, none of the patients showed spreading of cancer to other parts of the body. They also experienced no weight loss and less pain, and after twenty-four months, none of the women had died.

Take 90 mg of coenzyme Q10 in combination with the other nutrients listed. In cases of advanced cancer, higher therapeutic doses have been used.

## Calcium D-Glucarate (D-Glucaric Acid)

This compound is naturally found in foods like apples, Brussels sprouts, broccoli, cabbage, and bean sprouts. Studies show that taking D-glucarate prompts a slow release of a substance that inhibits glucuronidase, an enzyme that prevents the body from ridding itself of cancer-causing substances. Seventy percent of rats given a breast cancer-inducing chemical that were also pretreated with dietary glucarate did not develop tumors. The trial also discovered that glucarate lowered blood levels of estradiol (the form of estrogen most strongly linked to breast cancer). Researchers at M.D. Anderson Cancer Center, Memorial Sloan-Kettering Cancer Center, and other major cancer centers are conducting research on calcium D-glucarate for the prevention and treatment of breast cancer. Keep in mind, however, that no human studies showing the efficacy of calcium D-glucarate have been published to date.

Take 200–400 mg daily.

## Herbal Polysaccharides

Polysaccharides, the scientific name given to various complex "sugar" compounds, can initiate immune chain reactions that lead to improved immune function. There are numerous studies supporting the abilities of these sugars, or saccharides, to combat cancer, infections and other diseases. These sugars are largely found in various plants and herbs. Some of these include:

• aloe vera
• cordyceps sinensis
• coriolus mushroom
• echinacea
• astragalus
• reishi mushroom
• shiitake mushroom

## Daily Multivitamin-mineral and Antioxidant Mix

Taking a daily vitamin-mineral supplement is an easy, yet basic step in arming your body with the necessary nutrients. I also strongly recommend taking an array of antioxidants, especially if you are undergoing chemo or radiation. See Chapter 15 for my thoughts on antioxidants.

## Exercise and Ovarian Cancer

☐ ■ ■ ■

The benefits of movement are once again brought home by new findings that women who stay highly active throughout their lives are less likely to develop ovarian cancer. In this study, more than twenty-one hundred women were studied and those who exercised more than six hours per week were almost 30 percent less likely to develop ovarian cancer than women who exercised less than one hour per week. Not surprisingly, other studies show similar benefits for breast cancer as well. There is no question that regular exercise protects women of all ages from gynecological cancers, yet less than one fourth of women engage in regular physical activity. Which group do you belong to?

# Dietary Recommendations for Cancer Patients

*Avoid Alcohol.* Alcohol consumption has been linked to a higher risk of breast cancer, apparently because it raises estrogen levels.

*Increase Your Intake of Folic Acid.* Make sure you eat plenty of foods containing folic acid, which is shown to help prevent cancer. The best sources are dark green, leafy vegetables, such as spinach, chard, turnip greens, and broccoli, legumes, and orange juice.

*Eat Cruciferous Vegetables.* These include cauliflower, cabbage, broccoli and Brussels sprouts. Cruciferous vegetables contain a substance called indole-3-carbinol (I3C), which affects the way estrogen is metabolized. These vegetables also contain diindolyl-methane, which may also protect breast tissue. Numerous studies suggest that the higher your intake of vegetables, the lower your risk of breast cancer (a 25 percent decreased risk, in fact). Some experts argue that the data is flawed and that there's no proof that a high-vegetable/fruit diet lowers your risk. To them I say, "baloney." Take tomatoes, for example. They contain lycopene—an antioxidant that resembles beta-carotene. Several studies indicate that higher levels of lycopene correlate with a reduced risk of several types of cancer. Indoles and lycopene are also available in supplement form.

*Increase Your Fiber Intake.* Insoluble fiber found in whole grains puts women at a lower risk for female-related cancers. Why? Because it lowers estrogen levels and contains phytate and isoflavones, both of which protect breast tissue. New animal studies now confirm that IP-6 has anticancer activity. IP-6 (also called inositol hexaphosphate, phytate, or phytic acid) is found in oat bran, wheat bran, and unleavened bread.

Eat brown rice instead of white rice. Look for foods made with 100 percent whole grains. Eat raw nuts, legumes, and beans. Of course, most vegetables and fruits are fairly high in dietary fiber (and keep their skins on).

*Avoid Red Meat.* When compared with individuals who regularly eat meat, vegetarians have a lower risk of all kinds of cancer. Furthermore, they have more efficient immune systems (which, again, is ultimately the best weapon against any disease). In addition, vegetarian women have lower circulating estrogen levels compared with meat-eating women.

If you do eat meat, avoid charred or burned meats. Well-done meat contains more carcinogens than lightly cooked meat and some studies put women who eat overcooked meat at a higher risk of breast cancer.

*Try Fish!* Women who regularly eat fish have a 6 percent decreased risk of breast cancer. This is mostly due to the rich content of omega-3 fatty acids found in coldwater fish like salmon and tuna.

***Quit Coffee.*** While the jury is still out on coffee's relation to breast cancer, it has been linked to increased breast pain and may worsen fibrocystic breast disease. Many experts believe that women with fibrocystic breasts may also be more vulnerable to breast cancer. We do know that the caffeine in coffee can elevate estrogen levels, which may raise your risk of hormone-driven cancers.

***Use Extra Virgin Olive Oil.*** Consuming extra virgin olive oil is directly associated with a reduced risk of breast cancer in several preliminary reports. Olive oil is a monounsaturated fat whose protective actions may explain why Mediterranean cultures have lower rates of some cancers. Many books give wonderful recipes and easy guidelines on using olive oil in your diet.

***Decrease Your Overall Dietary Fat Intake.*** Many studies indicate that the higher your fat intake, the more prone you are to certain cancers. Estrogen levels are also impacted by fat stores and when women go on a low-fat diet, the density of their breast tissue decreases. If you've had breast cancer, eating foods high in hydrogenated, saturated and trans fats is strongly discouraged. Margarine, red meat, bacon, sausage and the like will increase your chances of recurrence. To illustrate this, look at the geographical dispersal of breast cancer. Women who live in countries where meat, dairy and refined foods dominate the diet have a much higher rate of breast cancer than those groups whose diet is largely made up of vegetables, rice, soy and fish.

***Eat More Soy.*** As you already know, soy and its isoflavone content represent a powerful tool in fighting cancer. There are numerous studies, coupled with its use in various cultures for thousands of years, that demonstrate soy's health benefits. Asian women who frequently consume tofu show significantly lower risk of breast and other hormone-stimulated cancers.

Researchers at Nebraska's Creighton University School of Medicine in Omaha conducted a study which found that soy dramatically reduces the movement of cancer cells from one site to another. Among forty-five soy-fed mice, dietary supplementation of soy protein significantly decreased the spread of cancer and the number of tumors that developed. In addition, another study published in *Free Radical Research* describes genistein as the most powerful antioxidant isoflavone, followed by daidzein. (You know by now how I feel about antioxidants. Refer to Chapter 15 for more details.) While there is some data suggesting that soy might, under some circumstances, increase the risk of breast cancer, I strongly disagree. The bottom line is that soy and its isoflavones are powerful cancer-protective agents.

***Decrease Your Sugar Intake.*** There is an association between high intakes of refined sugar (sucrose) or sugar-laden foods and an increased risk of breast cancer, not to mention its direct link with obesity and diabetes and other conditions.

## Adopt an Anticancer Lifestyle

***Lose Weight.*** The cancer research community recognizes that being overweight increases your risk of postmenopausal breast cancer. In addition, the more fat stores you carry, the more estrogen you make, which increases your chances of hormone-related cancer.

***Exercise Regularly.*** Girls who engage in regular exercise are less likely to get breast cancer as adults. Women who exercise are also reported to have less risk of high-risk mammography patterns compared with women who don't exercise.

One way that exercise may protect breast tissue is by lowering blood levels of estrogen and/or helping maintain an ideal body weight. Moreover, if you have cancer, a doctor-approved regimen of exercise can relieve depression and anxiety. Studies suggest that women who burn 200 calories daily have a lowered risk for cancer overall. In exercise lingo, that translates to approximately 40 minutes of walking at 3.2 miles per hour.

*Quit Smoking.* Several studies link smoking and second-hand smoke to an increased risk of breast cancer. In fact, recent press releases report that smoking is now associated with a variety of cancers. Simply put, smoking wreaks havoc on the human body.

*Reduce Stress and Improve Your Mood.* Your psychological and emotional health can make a big difference in your fight against cancer. For instance, studies show that the risk of breast cancer recurrence is higher in women who battle depression or have been exposed to severely stressful events (death of a spouse, divorce, etc.). In fact, the risk is more than five times higher in these women. There are all kinds of ways to reduce stress and anxiety levels. Relaxation training, exercise, meditation, massage, yoga, group therapy, and even hypnosis can all be helpful.

---

## Best Case Scenario

After diagnosing Rose with ovarian cancer, I put her on a course of transfer factor and genistein before, during and after chemotherapy treatments. In time, her blood became positive for cancer cells but there is absolutely no evidence of cancer anywhere in her body. And so, we continue with the protocol, which is designed to maximize her own immune defenses.

Chapter 12

□ ▨ ▪ ▨

# Osteoporosis: Facts and Fiction

If I knew I was going to live this long, I would have
taken better care of myself.
*– Unknown*

**More than eight** million American women have osteoporosis, and
it's estimated that another eighteen million will likely develop the
disease in the near future. These statistics are even more disturbing when you consider that by 2011, more than 25 percent of
Americans—a record number—will be older than fifty and at
high risk for developing this dangerous bone disease.

Osteoporosis gradually robs bones of their mineral reserves,
making them porous and weak, often years before symptoms surface. I've seen women whose bones were so brittle that even normal daily activities like lifting something heavy or turning over in
bed resulted in a bone fracture. Keep in mind that the hip, spine
and wrist are especially vulnerable. Although anyone can develop
osteoporosis, menopausal and postmenopausal women have the
highest risk. Osteoporosis is rarely seen in children and teenagers,
and men account for less than a quarter of osteoporosis cases
(they have higher bone densities than women). Even if a woman

hasn't been diagnosed with osteoporosis, she may still be losing bone mass (called osteopenia) and be well on her way to developing the disease. In fact, nearly half of all menopausal women have osteoporosis or osteopenia.

A broken bone may not seem like a big deal, but osteoporosis-related fractures are a serious health risk and often lead to disability and death among elderly women. It's estimated that one-third of older women will suffer a disabling hip fracture, and twenty of those women will die within a year of the fracture. Moreover, osteoporosis-related fractures, which average 1.5 million per year, account for $13.8 billion in hospital and nursing home costs each year—and those costs are going up. Osteoporosis can also cause long-term pain, deformity, reduced mobility, and breathing difficulties (if the ribs or back are seriously affected). Depression is a common consequence of the disease, since many victims suffer from isolation and a loss of independence.

No one knows exactly what causes osteoporosis, but decreased hormone production (estrogen in women, testosterone in men) and inadequate calcium in the diet are certainly involved. Your race and family history of the disease determine your risk. But so does your diet and physical activity. Remember that your bone mass status in your twenties and thirties also impacts what happens later. In other words, many circumstances that predispose a woman to osteoporosis are preventable, which means that despite what you may think, osteoporosis is not an inevitable consequence of aging.

## When Does Bone Loss Start?

You don't have to be menopausal to start losing bone density. In fact, by the time you get to menopause, you may have already lost considerable bone mass. You see, in healthy individuals bone is constantly being broken down and rebuilt. Before the age of thirty, the rate at which new bone is created is faster than the rate that existing bone is broken down. By the time a woman is fifty years old, however, bone mass breaks down faster than it can be replaced. Although the rate of bone loss varies, it can be as high as a 6 percent loss per year, especially in the years just after menopause.

Let me stress that if a young woman fails to achieve an ideal peak bone mass by the time she's thirty, she can develop osteoporosis at a younger age because her bone mass is already below average. In fact, a University of Arkansas study found that 2 percent of college-aged female participants already had osteoporosis and another 15 percent had significant osteopenia. This suggests that millions of young women are on their way to developing osteoporosis decades before symptoms appear. The greatest bone risks were found in young women using Depo-Provera (a form of birth control), those with low body weight or anorexia, and those who didn't consume enough dietary calcium (less than 50 percent of girls between the ages of nine and twelve consume enough calcium each day). In addition, young women who experience irregular periods or don't exercise regularly are also vulnerable to weaker bones.

## Symptoms of Osteoporosis

Osteoporosis can develop for years without symptoms. When symptoms emerge, they generally affect middle-aged or older women and include:

• back pain
• loss of height
• dowager's hump (a curved backbone)
• broken bones, especially in the hip, the spinal vertebrae and wrist

# Risk Factors for Osteoporosis

We've already talked briefly about some of the risk factors for osteoporosis, including age, gender, a family history of the disease, poor diet and poor exercise habits. Women with small frames, white and Asian women, and those with hormonal problems are also at risk. Let's take a closer look at some factors that may predispose you to osteoporosis.

## Ovarian Failure

According to a recent study published in *Obstetrics and Gynecology*, young women who constantly experience irregular periods (and aren't pregnant) may develop premature ovarian failure. The resulting hormonal shortage that accompanies this condition increases osteoporosis risk (estrogen is believed to help maintain bone density). According to the National Institutes of Health, roughly 1 percent of American women experience ovarian failure by age forty.

I know what you're probably thinking—what woman would complain about missing her period? Make no mistake—skipping periods can be a sign of other health problems and should be taken seriously enough to see your doctor. Although most women who skip the occasional period won't develop premature ovarian failure, 67 percent of women who do will also develop osteopenia. Unfortunately, many women with the disorder don't receive a proper diagnosis for years. A simple blood test for FSH (follicular stimulating hormone) can determine whether you suffer from premature ovarian failure. If you test positive for the condition, be sure to get your bone density checked as well. In simple terms, your ovaries produce the hormones that keep your bones flexible. When your menstrual cycle shuts down, it may signal ovarian failure—something that can't be ignored.

## Salt and Caffeine

Hide your salt shaker. Short-term increases in salt consumption may increase urinary calcium loss, which can cause bone loss over time. Although a concrete link between salt intake and osteoporosis has not yet been established, cutting down on your salt intake is wise, especially if you have high blood pressure or tend to retain water.

Caffeine is another culprit that increases urinary calcium loss and has been linked to a higher risk of hip fractures and lower bone mass, especially in women who don't consume adequate amounts of calcium. Too many women rely on caffeinated coffee and soft drinks to boost their energy levels. Caffeine may temporarily spike your energy levels, but it comes with a price. You can become dependent on its stimulation and feel like a deflated balloon when it wears off. Eating right and exercising are the only lasting ways to boost your energy reserves. The only exception appears to be caffeinated teas, which seem to prevent bone loss. Their bone-protective effects are probably due to their high phenol (antioxidant) content.

## Carbonated Drinks

Get rid of that forty-four-ounce soda sitting on your desk! Women who regularly consume carbonated soft drinks have an increased incidence of bone fractures. Soft drinks contain phosphoric acid, which impairs your body's ability to absorb or maintain calcium in the bones. Keep in mind that when phosphoric acid is absorbed, your blood can become more acidic. When this happens, built-in biological alarms go off and the body neutralizes the acid with alkaline materials like calcium and magnesium. Where does the calcium and magnesium come from? That's right, your bones. Soda often contains sodium as well, which can also weaken bone density.

Here's something to think about. Thirty years ago, our children drank twice as much milk as soda pop. By the mid-1990s, that statistic had reversed. Hard to believe, isn't it? Consequently, experts now have reason to believe that only 20 percent of our children consumes the minimum standard for calcium intake! To make matters worse, childhood years are the time when bone production is at an all-time high. As a result, these children may be more prone to bone fractures during adolescence and adulthood. In fact, more than one study suggests that teenage girls who drink more soda are more prone to broken bones. A 1994 Harvard study of bone fractures in teenage athletes found a strong association between soda beverage consumption and bone fractures in fourteen-year-old girls. The girls who drank soda were about five times more likely to suffer bone fractures than girls who didn't. The growing body of evidence indicating that young people have to worry about brittle bones or osteoporosis provides additional proof that the typical American diet is failing to protect our health, regardless of our age.

## Smoking

As if there aren't enough reasons to quit smoking, it is now believed that smoking also leads to increased bone loss. For instance, one study showed that women who smoke a pack of cigarettes a day lose 5 to 10 percent more bone density than nonsmokers by the time they reach menopause. Older women who smoke also have a 41 percent increase in the rate of hip fracture. Smoking reduces the blood supply to the bones, and nicotine inhibits the production of bone-forming cells (osteoblasts) and compromises calcium absorption. Smoking also appears to impair the actions of estrogen, which naturally protects bone mass. Bone density scanning is recommended for all women after the age of forty but is absolutely crucial if you smoke.

## Prescription Drugs

Several drugs can cause secondary osteoporosis, and if you are on any of them, talk to your doctor about preserving the health of your bones. If you must take one of these drugs, then for heaven's sake, take extra steps to protect your bones from additional damage. For instance, taking ipriflavone (a soy-derived supplement) may mitigate some of the bad effects of these drugs. Medications that pose the biggest threat include the following:

**Corticosteroids:** Cortisone, prednisone and dexamethasone are commonly prescribed corticosteroid drugs, and if used over a long period of time, pose a significant bone risk. The amount of bone loss you experience can vary depending on the type and form used. For instance, your bone loss may be greater if you take corticosteroids orally as opposed to using injections, inhalers or topical creams. Moreover, the stronger your dosage and the longer you take a corticosteroid drug, the higher your chances are for developing osteoporosis.

**Thyroid Hormone Drugs:** Most people who take this class of drug have an underactive thyroid. Because artificially manipulating this hormone can be tricky, an excessive dose can decrease bone mass over time. If you're on these drugs, make sure to have your blood thyroid levels tested every six months, and be diligent about taking calcium/magnesium supplements and exercising regularly.

**Antacids:** I don't recommend crunching on Tums to get your calcium. Tums are nothing more than calcium carbonate, a source of calcium that is not easily absorbed by the body. Antacid tablets containing aluminum should also be avoided—especially if you have kidney problems or repeatedly take them in high doses. The bottom line—don't rely on antacids as your only source of supplemental calcium. If you are using prescription antacid drugs, talk to your doctor about ways to counteract potential bone loss.

**Birth Control Pills:** Interestingly, some studies show that women who take birth control pills have lower bone mineral density (BMD) than women who have never used oral contraceptives. Data from a 2001 issue of the *Canadian Medical Association Journal* revealed that bone mineral density was up to 3.7 percent lower in women who used birth control pills compared with those who didn't. The bone loss appeared to target the spine and the upper part of the thigh bone. This effect may be the result of suppressed ovulation caused by the low doses of estrogen found in birth control pills. Depo-Provera, an injected form of birth control, has also been suspected of facilitating bone loss. Although some experts believe that using oral contraceptives may actually protect against osteoporosis by artificially elevating estrogen, there is enough conflicting data to make that belief suspect.

Other medications linked to bone loss include the following:

• phenytoin (Dilantin)
• barbiturates (used to prevent seizures)
• methotrexate (Rheumatrex, Immunex, Folex PFS)
• cyclosporine (Sandimmune, Neoral)
• luteinizing hormone-releasing hormone agonists (Lupron, Zoladex)
• heparin (Calciparine, Liquaemin)
• cholestyramine (Questran) and colestipol (Colestid)

# Conventional Treatment for Osteoporosis

Although many doctors recommend calcium supplements and regular weight-bearing exercise to women with osteoporosis,

## A Hormonal Quandary

□ ■ ■ ■

When it comes to bone health, higher estrogen levels usually enable more calcium to enter the bone matrix helping to preserve bone density. However, high circulating estrogen puts vulnerable tissue in the breast and other areas at risk for cancer. Interestingly, women who have breast cancer are less likely to develop osteoporosis, and women with osteoporosis have a lower risk of breast cancer. Can you see the estrogen link here? It's a catch twenty-two. But by using estrogen blockers like isoflavones and natural progesterone cream, a woman can have cancer *and* bone protection. It's like having your cake and eating it, too.

the most common medical solutions for serious cases include pharmaceuticals. Doctors often prescribe "designer estrogens" like raloxifene (Evista) to suppress the breakdown of bone, a nasal spray with calcitonin (Calcimar, Miacalcin) to prevent fractures, or bisphosphonates (Actonel) or alendronate (Fosamax) to reverse bone loss. Many of these drugs come with unpleasant side effects, so discuss all of your options with your doctor before deciding on a treatment. Unless your situation is extreme, nondrug alternatives may be your best bone-protecting option.

## Does HRT Prevent Osteoporosis?

Postmenopausal women are routinely encouraged to use hormone replacement therapy—e.g., estradiol (Estrace, Estraderm, FemPatch), conjugated estrogens (Premarin), and conjugated estrogens with medroxyprogesterone acetate (Premphase,

## Experimental Solutions for Bone Loss

□ ▪ ■ ■

A study which recently appeared in the October issue of *Science* suggests that a compound called estren (an estrogen-like drug) increased bone density and strength in mice with artificially induced menopause. The scientists also found that the compound had none of the dangerous side effects linked to estrogen. Estren is made from synthetic steroids and looks promising, but it's far from being ready for human consumption. Obviously, more research and testing are needed to determine its long-term effects and safety.

Prempro)—to halt bone loss. In fact, many women are told by their doctors that if they don't use HRT, they will almost definitely get osteoporosis. Yet only 6 percent of women in Japan use HRT, and according to some studies, Asian women have a significantly lower risk of osteoporosis compared with women who live in westernized countries. (Asian women living in the United States and eating western diets aren't so lucky.) Why do these women—who don't eat much dairy—have a lower risk of osteoporosis than American women? It's certain that they aren't wearing Depo patches or popping Provera.

While your doctor may protest, there is abundant research showing that synthetic hormones do *not* prevent bone loss. In fact, one study concluded that the risk of hip fractures for women over seventy-five is the same for those who took synthetic estrogen and those who didn't. Yes, studies also exist linking HRT to bone protection—the question is whether its potential benefits are worth the risk.

Here we go again. I believe that the most important aspect of osteoporosis management is its prevention. The higher your bone mass before menopause, the less your risk of osteoporosis later on. And good bones are not the result of HRT. Bone health depends on exercise and diet (surprise, surprise). Although the ability of estrogen to prevent osteoporosis still engenders debate, we do know this—synthetic estrogen *cannot* increase bone mass. Granted, it may delay or slow bone loss, but it can never replace bone. More importantly, conventional HRT comes with significant health risks that, more often than not, outweigh any bone-protective benefits.

## Bone Density and Soy Isoflavones

Although no long-term human studies have definitively linked soy isoflavones to higher bone density or low fracture risk, research looks promising. Researchers at the University of Illinois in Urbana found that soy isoflavones can help to strengthen the bones of the lumbar spine and help to prevent the dowager's hump often seen in postmenopausal women with osteoporosis. The bone density of one group of women who took 92 mg of soy isoflavones daily increased by 2.2 percent over a period of six months.

In another double-blind trial, postmenopausal women who consumed 40 grams of soy protein powder (containing 90 mg of isoflavones) per day were protected against bone mineral loss in the spine, although lower amounts were not found to be protective. Perhaps most convincing are the findings of another study which observed that women using genistein retained the same bone mineral mass as those using prescription doses of estradiol. How many women on traditional HRT know that?

Bone loss in women appears to coincide with drops in estrogen. The isoflavones found in soy can naturally boost declining estrogen levels. Eating soy foods such as tofu, soy milk, roasted soy beans, and soy protein powders is a good way to get these much-needed isoflavones. Additionally, some scientists believe that genistein inhibits the action of osteoclasts (cells that work to remove bone tissue). Soy is also a good source of calcium—one serving of tofu can contain 120–750 mg of calcium.

Unlike meat, the protein found in soy is bone friendly. Studies show that certain amino acids in animal proteins impair calcium absorption. Research also reveals that animal protein consumption causes more calcium to be excreted from the body, thereby weakening bone mass. Soy protein and other vegetable proteins do not appear to have this effect. One study found that diets of all animal protein averaged calcium excretions of 150 mg a day, while excretions from those on soy protein diets were a third lower.

Most women lose 2–3 percent of bone density in the two to three years following menopause. Consuming soy before and after this crucial period may significantly reduce osteoporosis risk. In fact, women in their twenties and thirties should consider using soy for bone protection, since these are critical years for developing maximum bone mass.

## Ipriflavone: Potentiated Isoflavone Compound for Bone Health

Ipriflavone is an isoflavone synthesized from daidzein, which is naturally found in soy. It appears to have significant potential in the prevention and treatment of osteoporosis and other bone diseases. Although it has no estrogenic activity itself, it safely boosts the effect of estrogen. Studies have found that it enhances bone formation and mineral absorption, thereby increasing bone density. Ipriflavone has the distinct ability to increase the activity of bone-building cells called osteoblasts while simultaneously inhibiting the action of osteoclasts (which actually break down bone material). One study conducted in 1998 found that ipriflavone was able to dramatically boost new bone formation and repair. A group of fifty-six postmenopausal women with low bone density all received 1,000 mg of calcium and random subjects were given an additional 600 mg of ipriflavone. The women who took only calcium experienced increased bone loss after two years. By contrast, bone loss was totally halted in those who also took ipriflavone. The study concluded that 600 mg of ipriflavone taken daily prevents the rapid bone loss following early menopause.

Preliminary data shows that ipriflavone may be especially helpful for those who use corticosteroids, are immobile, or have had their ovaries removed. For this reason, if osteoporosis runs in your family but you're concerned about the safety of conventional HRT, ipriflavone may be a good choice for you.

## Progesterone Stimulates Bone Production

While I heartily believe that soy can protect bone, I think that the addition of progesterone makes for even more powerful bone protection. There is plenty of evidence suggesting that progesterone preserves bone mass and stimulates the production of bone, thereby reducing osteoporosis risk. In fact, one study published in the *Journal of Bone and Mineral Research* concluded that progesterone maintained the creation of bone, while discouraging bone breakdown. Researchers finished by saying, "These findings suggest that progesterone alone may be a valuable agent for management of postmenopausal osteoporosis." Apparently, progesterone is able to stimulate bone-building osteoblasts, which cannot be accomplished with HRT use. I believe that complementing soy with natural progesterone cream for bone health is a great idea.

## Take the Right Calcium Supplement

Close to three quarters of all women *don't* get enough calcium in their diets, and over 50 percent don't even get half the recommended amount. In addition, women who are allergic to milk, lactose-intolerant or avoiding dairy for weight loss may be more at risk for calcium depletion. Unfortunately, you may not find out that you're calcium deficient until your teeth and bones start falling apart.

The good news is that calcium supplements are a good way to ensure that you get enough calcium, and they are relatively inexpensive. The bad news? Choosing the right kind is often tricky and confusing. Many women think that the more calcium a product has, the better. Not so. What counts is how much calcium is actually absorbed into the bones.

There are three commonly available forms of this mineral—calcium carbonate, calcium lactate and calcium citrate. According to the latest research, calcium citrate wins over its competitors for absorbability. A study in the November 1999 issue of the *Journal of Clinical Pharmacology* revealed that the human body absorbs two-and-a-half times more calcium citrate than calcium carbonate. So while calcium carbonate supplements may contain more elemental calcium than calcium citrate, less of it actually finds its way into your bones.

If your calcium supplement contains multiple types of calcium, make sure that calcium citrate is the top ingredient. Also, avoid calcium supplements derived from bone meal, oyster shell or dolomite. These supplements may be contaminated with lead. And if you have kidney disease, kidney stones or an overactive parathyroid gland, you should check with your doctor before taking any calcium supplement.

## Maximizing the Action of a Calcium Supplement

• Choose a calcium supplement that contains vitamin D and magnesium to enhance its absorption. The calcium-magnesium ratio in the supplement you choose should be two-to-one (for example, 500 mg calcium to 250 mg magnesium).

• If possible, spread your calcium doses throughout the day, limiting each dose to no more than 500 mg. This helps to increase absorption and decrease any possible side effects, which can include constipation and bloating.

• Take your supplement with a large glass of water to ensure that it breaks down properly, or use chewable calcium tablets, powders or liquids. The last thing you need is a bunch of undissolved calcium tablets hiding in your colon. Don't take calcium supplements with meals because dietary fiber can bind with calcium and prevent its absorption.

## Minimum Calcium Requirements

• Premenopausal women: 1,000–1,200 mg daily
• Pregnant/nursing women: 1,200–1,500 mg daily
• Postmenopausal women under age sixty-five (on estrogen replacement therapy): 1,000–1,200 mg daily
• Postmenopausal women under age sixty-five (not on estrogen replacement therapy): 1,500 mg daily
• All women over age sixty-five: 1,200–1,500 daily

My recommendation is that most individuals can safely take up to 2,000 mg/day of calcium, but I believe the ideal dose is between 1,200 and 1,500 mg of calcium citrate each day.

## Dairy Products—Bone Friend or Foe?

England, Australia and the United States have the highest rates of osteoporosis. Is it just a coincidence that citizens of these countries also eat the most dairy products and red meat? I know what you're thinking—don't milk, cheese and other dairy products provide much needed calcium for bone strength? Perhaps not. Several theories suggest that pasteurized and artificially treated milk and cheese are not digested the way they should be; therefore, their calcium content may not be adequately absorbed. Moreover, diets high in animal protein (from meat and dairy) are not bone friendly. Certain amino acids found in these proteins may cause calcium to be leached from your bones and teeth.

If you're going to consume dairy products, choose nonfat milk, which has a lower protein and salt content, but sports a higher calcium content. Cottage cheese is not a good choice because it's actually higher in protein and salt, and lower in calcium. Many hard cheeses are also high in fat and salt and are not preferable sources of dietary calcium. Low-fat yogurt offers another good source of dietary calcium, but make sure to choose products with "active" lactobacteria cultures.

# How to Prevent and Even Reverse Bone Loss

## Eat More Vegetables

You already know my views on how we should eat, but consider this. A recent study in the *Journal of Clinical Nutrition* conducted at the University of California Medical School in San Francisco emphasized the importance of maintaining a proper balance between the consumption of animal protein and vegetable protein for bone health. Researchers found that menopausal women whose protein consumption was three-to-one (favoring animal protein over vegetable protein) had a much higher risk of osteoporosis and hip fractures. When that ratio dropped to one-to-one, the risk dramatically dropped.

---

### Preferred Calcium-Rich Foods

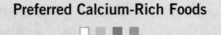

- nonfat and low-fat dairy, including active culture yogurt and milk
- dark green, leafy vegetables, such as broccoli, kale and collards
- canned sardines and salmon with edible bones
- calcium-fortified orange juice and cereal
- tofu and soymilk
- raw almonds

---

Another study found that women who were vegetarians for at least twenty years have an average mineral bone loss of 18 percent. By comparison, meat-eating women lost 35 percent of their bone mineral content. Moreover, many vegetables are rich in vitamin K, which works to maintain calcium deep within your bones. While you may find opposing arguments by other experts, I believe that obtaining your protein from soy and other legumes (beans, raw nuts, etc.) is not only bone protective, but is much better for your entire body. As opposed to red meat and dairy products, when was the last time you saw red beans or almonds linked to heart disease or cancer? And I must add that my vegetarian patients have excellent bone mass and flexibility. In virtually every health category, they far surpass my "meat-and-potato" patients.

### Choose Your Oils Wisely

Amazingly, in one study, elderly women with osteoporosis who were given 4 grams of fish oil per day for four months had improved calcium absorption and even showed evidence of new bone formation. Combing fish oil with evening primrose oil (EPO) may be even better. In another controlled study, women who took 6 grams of a combination of EPO and fish oil plus 600 mg of calcium per day for three years experienced no spinal bone loss in the first eighteen months and showed a dramatic 3.1 percent increase in spinal bone mineral density during the last eighteen months.

You can take EPO and fish oils in capsule form, and I like to add vitamin E to the mix.

## Magnify Your Magnesium

If you have osteoporosis, you may also have trouble absorbing magnesium. Low blood and bone levels of this mineral are frequently found in women suffering from osteoporosis. In a two-year, controlled trial, magnesium supplementation at 250 mg to 750 mg per day actually stopped bone loss or increased bone mass in 87 percent of people with osteoporosis. You need to take a minimum of 350 mg of magnesium with your calcium daily.

## Vitamin D for Density

Good ol' vitamin D boosts calcium absorption. Your blood levels of this vital vitamin are directly related to the strength of your bones. A deficiency of vitamin D is common in elderly women and accelerates age-related bone loss and increases fracture risk. Many studies show that vitamin D supplementation reduces bone loss in women who don't get enough of it in their diets. Dietary sources of vitamin D include eggs, fatty fish such as sardines, and milk and cereal fortified with vitamin D. Exposure to twenty minutes of sunlight each day also boosts vitamin D levels. Women between the ages of nineteen and fifty should aim for 200 IU of vitamin D each day, and for women aged fifty-one to seventy, 400 IU is recommended. Women older than seventy should get 600 IU of vitamin D each day.

## Include Vitamin K

Women who have osteoporosis are also frequently low in vitamin K. One study found that postmenopausal women can actually decrease their urinary calcium loss by taking 1 mg of vitamin K per day. Among women who already have osteoporosis, supplementation with vitamin K increases bone density and decreases bone loss after six months.

## Look for Trace Minerals

Trace minerals like zinc and copper are also critical for proper bone mass, and chelated forms should be included in your vitamin and mineral supplement. You should be getting 10 mg of zinc and 2–3 mg of copper daily.

## Start Young

Encourage your teenage daughters to develop healthy bone habits early, including taking calcium supplements, eating right and exercising regularly. The best time to build strong bones is during the second decade of life. Research demonstrates that twelve-year-old girls who took calcium supplements had better bone building capabilities than those who did not. The more bone mass you can build when you're young, the less your risk of osteoporosis later.

## Lose Weight

Someone told one of my overweight patients that she had a lower risk of osteoporosis because fat cells make estrogen. Although that assumption was technically correct, too much extra weight stresses your bones and muscles and is ultimately not bone healthy. Moreover, obese women are at higher risk for breast cancer, heart disease, diabetes and other health problems.

If you lose weight the right way—with a healthy diet and regular weight-bearing exercise—you will fare better in all respects. And the sooner you begin these healthy habits, the better.

## Engage in Weight-Bearing Exercise

Engaging in weight-bearing exercises is an absolute must for sustained bone health. Women who exercise at least three times a week consistently show higher bone mineral content than those who don't. Weight-bearing exercise stimulates the growth of bone and muscle tissue, strengthens the skeleton and reduces osteoporosis and arthritis risk as well. Any activity that involves resistance, i.e. pushing, lifting or carrying a heavy object, is considered weight-bearing exercise. This includes walking, jogging, water and step aerobics, free weights, exercise balls and bands and resistance machines. Mild weightlifting can be helpful, but you should avoid exercises that put an abnormal amount of stress on your bones and joints. Simply stated, regular exercise protects against bone loss, and the more weight-bearing exercise you do, the better your bone mass will be.

□ ▨ ■ ▨

# Chapter 13

# The Little-Known Hysterectomy Alternative

*When in doubt, cut it out; a chance to cut is a chance to cure.*
*– Surgeon's credo*

**America has the** dubious distinction of leading the world in hysterectomies. Over six hundred thousand hysterectomies are performed on American women each year, and approximately half of all women will be without a uterus by the time they are sixty-five. In the state of Utah alone, hysterectomy is the most common surgical procedure by a factor of four (after cesarean section). Yet it's estimated that less than 50 percent of all hysterectomies are justified. What's behind these outrageous statistics?

One reason is that many doctors don't know any better. They are in what I call a "surgical rut"—still holding on to outdated views that they learned in medical school. Some medical textbooks still allude to hysterectomy as the "end all" surgery for women. A few swift turns of the scalpel and the offending parts are gone—and everyone lives happily ever after. In reality, a hysterectomy is an easier solution for the surgeon. Taking out a whole system of organs requires little finesse. It's much more challenging and time consuming for a physician to find alternatives to wholesale organ removal.

For years, women incorrectly diagnosed with cervical cancer and advised to have a hysterectomy have come to see me for a second opinion. And more than once after performing a colposcopy, I discovered they didn't have cancer to begin with. I know of three women in their twenties who almost lost their reproductive organs based on a false cancer diagnosis. I was able to remove their cervical abnormalities with surgery, and all three women were later able to have children. In fact, they all still "own" a uterus and are now well into their menopausal years.

Don't get me wrong. Sometimes a hysterectomy is a good idea, and when it is, I'm all for it. If a woman has a seriously prolapsed uterus, cancer, uncontrollable bleeding or extremely large fibroids, removing her reproductive organs can greatly improve the quality of her life. However, I've found that heavy or irregular menstrual bleeding, the presence of small uterine fibroids, mild pelvic relaxation and abnormal Pap smears can lead to hysterectomies that should have never happened. Of equal importance, many doctors view a hysterectomy as an inconsequential surgery. It's anything but that. Of the five to six hundred thousand hysterectomies performed annually, complications are noted in 35 percent of cases. Moreover, over 600 women die from this "simple procedure" annually. Even if a woman makes a full recovery from the surgery, she can suffer from a number of side effects. Unfortunately, when a doctor tells you that you need a hysterectomy, he rarely discusses what you can expect post-op.

## Side Effects Associated with a Hysterectomy

• anxiety
• bone loss

• bowel and bladder complications
• depression
• headaches
• increased risk of heart disease
• joint and muscle aches
• lethargy
• pelvic pain
• sexual problems (painful intercourse, etc.)
• skin changes
• weight gain

# Why It's Good to Hold onto Your Ovaries

The removal of any healthy organ should always be avoided if possible. Removing a woman's ovaries can drastically influence her health. And even if they are left in after a hysterectomy, the inevitable disruption of blood flow can eventually render them useless, which explains why ovarian cysts often occur after a hysterectomy. Ovaries do much more than hold eggs. They are a woman's primary source of hormones (estrogen, progesterone and a small amount of testosterone). For too many doctors, preserving a woman's ovaries for as long as possible takes a back seat to "getting it all" in one clean sweep.

Even if you had a hysterectomy and kept your ovaries, you may not know for some time that you have become estrogen deficient. If you're young, you may not experience any of the typical symptoms associated with menopause. Symptoms or not, without estrogen you are at a much higher risk for heart disease and osteoporosis. Even at a young age, your bones will steadily lose their calcium content.

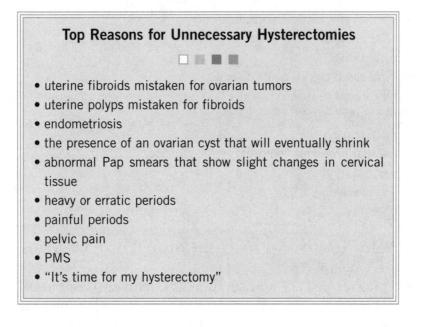

**Top Reasons for Unnecessary Hysterectomies**

- uterine fibroids mistaken for ovarian tumors
- uterine polyps mistaken for fibroids
- endometriosis
- the presence of an ovarian cyst that will eventually shrink
- abnormal Pap smears that show slight changes in cervical tissue
- heavy or erratic periods
- painful periods
- pelvic pain
- PMS
- "It's time for my hysterectomy"

## A Typical Scenario

I recently saw Marcia, a forty-six-year-old mother who wanted a second opinion after being advised to have a hysterectomy. Her only complaints were PMS, breast tenderness and irregular spotting (symptoms of estrogen dominance), but she was reluctant to try hormones due to her family's strong history of breast cancer. Her primary-care physician reasoned that she should have her uterus removed while she was still healthy since she would inevitably require a hysterectomy in the future. After our consultation, I placed Marcia on genistein and natural progesterone cream to resolve her estrogen overload. As a result, she now has light, regular periods without PMS and breast tenderness. She also noted an unexpected increase in her libido. Marcia is one of a long list of women in my practice who avoided going under the knife by using alternative treatments.

# Get "In the Know"

The approach I just described has been used successfully by hundreds of women with excellent results and supports the notion (also backed by numerous studies) that very few women should have a hysterectomy because of bleeding problems or other symptoms of estrogen dominance. Excessive or irregular menstrual bleeding is more often than not caused by a hormone imbalance, and in most instances can be treated medically, not surgically. Before she considers a hysterectomy for menstrual cycle problems, a woman should first try regular exercise, dietary changes and the dynamic duo—genistein and natural progesterone cream. More often than not, these approaches make a hysterectomy unnecessary.

Women with heavy periods are also prime candidates for another little-known hysterectomy alternative, a technique I developed called rollerball or endometrial ablation (in use since 1988). Some women continue to suffer from heavy or irregular periods regardless of supplemental therapy or dietary changes. If you fall into this category, you may opt for this procedure.

# Endometrial Ablation: Lose the Lining, Keep the Organ

Endometrial ablation is a term used to describe the destruction of the endometrium (the lining of the uterus). If you eliminate endometrial cells, they no longer build up and shed each month. The best part about endometrial ablation is that it stops (or greatly reduces) menstrual bleeding without removing the uterus. The result of the procedure is either very light periods or no periods at all. It can be done in a variety of ways and ultimately saves many women from having a hysterectomy.

It's important not to confuse an endometrial ablation with

having a "D&C" (affectionately referred to as a "dusting and cleaning," or more accurately "dilation and curettage"), where the uterine lining is scraped. This procedure is a hit-and-miss proposition which can skip large areas of the endometrium. Moreover, it only affects the immediate surface of the uterine lining. Ablation goes much deeper.

### Heavy Periods at Fifty

The first time Judy saw me for a consultation, she was fifty years old and suffered from PMS, heavy bleeding, weight gain, low libido and mood disorders. Her primary-care physician put her on birth control pills (as they most often do), making her even more miserable. She began suffering from bloating and headaches. Her doctor told her that if the hormones didn't work, she would need a total hysterectomy. A gynecologist confirmed the primary-care physician's opinion—her only choice was a hysterectomy with removal of her ovaries. Neither doctor mentioned two other viable options: ablation of the uterine lining and supplementation with genistein and natural progesterone cream.

After spending some time talking with Judy and taking a thorough history, it became obvious that she was estrogen dominant. Estrogen dominance is not a justifiable cause for a hysterectomy. We placed her on genistein and natural progesterone, which took care of most of her symptoms. Later, I treated a fibroid tumor in her uterine cavity with endometrial ablation. Judy continues to use genistein and natural progesterone. Today, she feels "wonderful"—and she still owns her uterus and ovaries.

## Endometrial Ablation Methods

• Using the Yag Laser to destroy the lining of the uterus; this method takes up to four times longer than using the rollerball technique.

• Using very hot water to "cook" the uterine lining; the results are not as good as those using the rollerball technique, and the extreme heat can cause considerable post-operative pain.

• Using microwaves and electrical currents to destroy the lining; while short-term results look good, long-term data supporting these procedures is lacking.

• Using an electric cautery ball or rollerball to eliminate the lining (rollerball endometrial ablation).

• Freezing the lining of the uterus (cryoablation), now considered the safest method, and one that can be performed in a physician's office.

## The Rollerball Option

The rollerball technique uses a ball-shaped electrode that delivers energy to the uterine lining and by so doing, destroys the endometrium. Not only does the rollerball technique efficiently cover the lining, it can also be used to seal off or cauterize the wall of the uterus after the lining is destroyed. While most methods of ablation work, the rollerball procedure is one of the most effective. By opting for the rollerball, you spend less time on the operating table, which decreases the cost of the operation and potential risks. In fact, it's an out-patient procedure and doesn't require hospitalization.

Keep in mind, however, that endometrial ablation is not appropriate for younger women who desire to have children or women who have uterine cancer. The procedure usually causes sterility, although a small portion of uterine lining may remain intact, making it possible to conceive. I advise women having an ablation to get a tubal ligation at the same time, since post-ablation pregnancies have substantial complications. Otherwise, the risks of this procedure are few and rare. Because a large volume of fluid is used during the surgery, alteration in blood elec-

## The Fibroid Solution

◻ ▪ ▪ ▪

Fibroids and polyps (sometimes referred to as "myomas") are commonly formed in the uterine cavity. They are non-cancerous growths that develop in the muscular tissue that lines the wall of the uterus. Fibroids are notorious for causing menstrual pain and heavy bleeding, although some women have no symptoms with fibroids. Your risk of fibroids increases until you reach menopause, and for unknown reasons, African-American women are at a higher risk for developing fibroids. It's estimated that up to half of these women have fibroids.

Due to unpleasant periods associated with fibroids, many women end up having a hysterectomy to remedy the problem. This disturbs me because in many cases, ablation is the best way to remove the majority of uterine fibroids and polyps. Cryoablation (the freezing technique) can remove fibroids that are as large as a small grapefruit. The closer you are to menopause when you have an ablation, the better your chances that they won't recur.

Interestingly, I recently returned from a seminar in Rome where an Italian gynecology specialist discussed the possibilities of using cryosurgery through a laparoscope to destroy the primary blood supply to fibroids. Regardless of the method of fibroid removal, using genistein and natural progesterone cream after the procedure is crucial to block estrogen receptors in uterine tissue. What stimulates the growth of fibroids? Estrogen. This specialist agreed with my assessment that excess estrogen helps to create fibroids and that blocking estrogen would help to prevent their recurrence.

trolytes can occur, and there is the rare possibility of puncturing the uterus. However, I consider the surgery extremely safe and effective. It is an infinitely better option than a hysterectomy.

# What to Expect Before and After Rollerball Ablation

The day before the surgery, a small piece of seaweed called *laminaria* is placed into the cervix to absorb moisture, causing the cervix to dilate. Some cramping is normal, but is usually well-controlled with over-the-counter pain medication. You will also be given a prescription for antibiotics (as a precaution) that you should take for three to five days after the procedure.

After the surgery, some women notice a brownish or slightly bloody vaginal discharge. This is perfectly normal and can occur off and on for several weeks. I advise women who have had an ablation to refrain from exercise for three weeks to ensure proper healing. Otherwise, side effects are minimal. Half of all women who have the procedure don't experience any side effects whatsoever. The other half may experience mild cramps for up to a week after the surgery. Most women can pretty much resume their normal routine after only a few days. In virtually every patient I've treated with ablation, the menstrual flow is dramatically reduced or ceases altogether, though it does take a year to adequately assess the final results. About 10 percent of women who have ablation will experience irregular episodes of spotting. If these persist, a second rollerball ablation may be necessary.

### Liz's New Lease on Life

Liz was in her late forties when her periods began to interfere with her life. She felt ill for days on end, and her periods were becoming heavier and more erratic. When they began to disrupt trips and other important events, she knew she had to do something. Liz was still a decade away from menopause, and couldn't cope with the prospect that these problems could continue for years.

After hearing about rollerball ablation, Liz decided to schedule an appointment with me. Although she hated medical procedures, she agreed to same-day surgery. Afterward, Liz felt a bit groggy, but she had no pain and no unpleasant side effects whatsoever. She couldn't believe how simple it was, and her periods have stopped completely. In a follow-up visit, she told me, "I feel ten years younger—I can't believe more women don't know about this!"

## A Crucial Follow-Up Treatment for Any Ablation

My prescription for success after an ablation differs somewhat from other gynecologists who do the procedure. To keep fibroids or the uterine lining from growing back, I tell my post-procedure patients to go on a regimen of genistein and natural progesterone supplementation for at least six months. Genistein works to block estrogen receptors in the uterus. Patients that have done so get essentially 100 percent control of their bleeding.

I also recommend periodic follow-up visits. During these visits, I not only check the progress of my patients, but also drill home the importance of using genistein and natural progesterone cream, adopting good eating habits, and developing an exercise regimen. Together, these habits are the key to preventing estrogen-driven endometrial regrowth, fibroids and other symptoms. They also reduce breast and uterine cancer risks. Women who take my advice seriously have a phenomenal rate of post-op success and are less likely to need secondary ablations.

## The Fast Freeze

□ ■ ■ ■

As popular as rollerball ablation is, I think the best all-around method of ablation is cryoablation, or "the fast freeze." It utilizes intense cold to destroy the uterine lining (in much the same way that it eradicates precancerous lesions of the uterine cervix). During cryoablation, I use ultrasound technology to monitor my progress in real time. Consequently, it is the only method currently available that has the best likelihood of success. Plus, since cold has an analgesic effect, cryoablation is often performed in the physician's office with minimal pain. I use a local anesthetic, and there is virtually no downtime after the procedure. Many women tell me that they experienced *no* pain during and after the ablation, and it's exceptionally safe as well.

Although I introduced rollerball ablation and have used it with nearly two thousand women, I currently lean toward cryoablation because of its simplicity, safety and effectiveness. And when combined with genistein and natural progesterone therapy, it results in a 90 percent success rate. An added bonus is that cryoablation is easier to teach to other physicians.

# Spreading the Word

Years ago, the remarkable advantages of uterine ablation came to the attention of a well-known actress who had tried virtually every known prescription drug to control her menstrual flow with no success. The actress was delighted with the results of her surgery and in 1989, was featured in an article for *Ladies Home Journal* on the merits of rollerball ablation. She said that at that point in her life, having a hysterectomy would have been like having an amputation. (In retrospect, I believe the actress had the classic symptoms of estrogen excess or dominance, of which I was still unaware. Consequently, I believe that using genistein and natural progesterone would have improved her results that much more!)

Shortly after the article appeared, we got calls from women all over North America. (I was the only physician doing the procedure at that time.) I received enough referrals to keep me busy for two years.

During the 1990s, I went on a nationwide tour to teach physicians the rollerball technique, and many came to me to learn. The word is getting out. Although this transfer of knowledge went on for over a decade, there are still thousands of women who remain unaware of the surgery and its advantages over a hysterectomy. Too many doctors don't explain hysterectomy alternatives to their patients, and HMO interference may also keep women in the dark.

## The Never-Ending Flow

Tina came to see me for intractable uterine bleeding due to the presence of fibroids. She was referred by a specialist who was open-minded enough to recommend alternative approaches to women who wanted to avoid unnecessary major surgery. The forty-six-year-old had been bleeding daily for over nine months and had tried several different hormone regimens without success. Her doctor told her to get a hysterectomy, but she told me that she was single-handedly running her own business and just couldn't take the time off. I offered her a rollerball ablation but even that didn't fit into her schedule. So I suggested that she try taking genistein and using natural progesterone cream, and somewhat reluctantly, she agreed.

In four weeks, Tina came into my office so I could check her progress. She confessed that she was initially very skeptical about my suggestion. She thought I might be a "witch doctor." I chuckled and asked her how she felt. She happily replied that the day after she started using the genistein and natural progesterone, she stopped bleeding and had not bled since. Six weeks later, she told me that she had a light, three-day period but no irregular bleeding or spotting. Eventually, Tina chose to have an ablation.

## Speak Up

Ultimately, it's up to you to ask the right questions if your doctor recommends a hysterectomy. Get a second or even third opinion before you make a decision. Any time you get any diagnosis from your gynecologist, scrutinize it. No one knows your body like you do. An excellent review of the consequences of hysterectomy can be found in the book *Hysterectomy and Ovary Removal*, by Elizabeth Ploudre. Take it with you to your appointment and insist that your doctor address some of the issues Ploudre brings up. Or check the Internet for websites, including my own (see the Resource section) that discuss the pro's and cons of hysterectomy. It can help to write down your alternatives. Become a pebble in your physician's shoe—keep asking questions until you're satisfied that you have all the facts. Most of all, if your doctor casts off your concerns, get another physician. If you are diligent, chances are you can avoid going under the knife.

Chapter 14

□ ▨ ■ ■

# Demystifying Vaginal and Vulvar Infections

*Medical scientists are nice people, but you should not let them treat you.*
*— August Bier (1861-1949) German surgeon*

**In 1979 I** went into private practice at Cedar Sinai Hospital in Beverly Hills. There, I met a physician from Houston named Carl Karnaky. Carl had a radical notion that vaginal yeast infections could be treated effectively without using topical antifungal creams (the conventional treatment). I was intrigued and asked him to show me his solution. He gave me a special powder he'd been using to make the vagina very acidic and unhospitable to yeast organisms causing the infection. I liked the acidifying powder so much that I began using it on my own patients.

When a woman would come in complaining of itching and vaginal discharge, I first evaluated her condition using a potassium hydroxide screening test, also called the "wet mount technique" (no fancy testing procedures were available yet). If she tested positive for a yeast infection, I would apply a dose of the fine, flour-like (and sometimes messy) powder to the area. Its application would inevitably cause a small cloud of white mist to float up from the end of the examining table. Unfortunately, although the powder worked wonderfully, it was virtually impossible to teach a patient how to use it herself. It was just too hard to handle.

So, we decided to use capsules of boric acid powder to acidify the vagina and it worked beautifully. The new method was also inexpensive, effective and easy for the patient to use. In fact, it costs no more than 40 cents per treatment, in contrast to expensive creams and prescriptions commonly used today. Acidification isn't just for yeast infections—it also helps eradicate bacterial infections of the vagina as well.

## Yeast Infections Are Common

Approximately 75 percent of all women will experience at least one yeast infection during their lifetimes. Vaginal yeast infections (vulvovaginal candidiasis) occur when the *Candida albicans* fungus (a natural inhabitant of the vaginal canal) overgrows. Several things can cause this proliferation of yeast including antibiotic use, diabetes, pregnancy, intercourse, hormonal changes, nutritional deficiencies and poor hygiene.

If you've had a yeast infection (and chances are you have) you're only too familiar with the symptoms—itching, burning, redness and a thick discharge. Always see a physician if you have any symptoms of a vaginal infection. Left untreated (or not fully treated), these infections can cause more serious problems. Furthermore, not all vaginal infections are caused by the candida yeast fungus. Another common infection, bacterial vaginosis, produces similar symptoms, and a vaginal infection may also be a sign of a sexually transmitted disease called trichomoniasis (the third most common cause of vaginal infection). Other STDs can cause vaginal symptoms similar to those of a yeast infection as well. Frequent yeast infections are sometimes a sign of health problems like diabetes or HIV infection.

# Oral Medications for Vaginal Infections: Putting the Horse Before the Cart

Have you seen the latest pharmaceutical campaign to treat yeast infections? The newest approach is to take oral antifungal pills to treat a localized yeast infection. The treatment is described as hassle-free. In other words, in order to avoid "messy applications," you can just pop a pill. The truth is, promoting oral medications for vaginal infections defies common sense. Instead of treating a localized problem with a topical medicine, these companies advocate sending a powerful antifungal chemical through the bloodstream that affects every organ in the body on its way to the vaginal canal (especially the liver).

This mentality is nothing less than an opportunistic ploy by pharmaceutical companies who want to increase their sales of drugs for vaginal infection. And they may succeed since vaginal creams are messy and inconvenient. This convoluted logic powerfully illustrates our obsession with any "magic pill" therapy and the marketing prowess of the pharmaceutical industry. They would have women taking a handful of drugs daily whether they needed them or not.

A single pill costs about ten times as much as using simple acidification. You may be thinking, "No problem, my insurance pays for the drugs." Don't you believe it! We all pay in the end with higher premiums. Yes, these pills do get rid of yeast infections, but they can also cause liver disease, and pregnant women using drugs for vaginal infections need to be especially careful. A new study shows that women taking the drug metronidazole (Flagyl) for a vaginal infection can go into premature labor. A startling 19 percent of the women who received the drug delivered their babies before thirty-seven weeks' gestation.

# How to Use Acidification

So why use acidification instead of over-the-counter creams to treat yeast infections? It's simple—acidification is just as effective and you don't need a medical degree to do it! Remember that antifungal preparations may contain antihistamines or topical anesthetics that only mask the symptoms of the infection and do nothing to treat the underlying cause. Acidification works, it's cheaper, it applies easy and is less messy than creams.

### What you need:
- One 4-ounce jar of boric acid powder at the drug store. Cost: $3–$4
- Thirty empty gelatin capsules from your health food store. Cost: $3–$4

### How to prepare the treatment:
- Pull apart about a dozen capsules and set them on a tabletop.
- Pour a small mound of boric acid powder into the cap from the boric acid bottle.
- Scoop the boric acid into both halves of the empty capsules, assemble and put the full capsules aside.

### Directions for applying the treatment:
- At the first sign of infection, insert one capsule high into the vagina twice daily each morning and night for one week. (For less severe infections, use only one capsule a day, inserted at night, for seven days.) If you notice any burning after insertion, empty 1/2 of the boric acid out of the next capsule, and use only 1/2 capsule of boric acid with each treatment. If you plan to have sex during treatment (not recommended during the first week since the infection can be transferred to your partner), insert the capsule after sexual relations.

• After one week, self-treat only at night (one capsule per day) for another week.

• For the third week, insert one capsule every third night.

• If desired, insert one capsule weekly for an indefinite period of time as a preventive treatment. This program can be repeated as necessary.

## Victory Over Vulvar Itching

Invariably, a woman with a vaginal infection experiences vulvar pruritus (itching), but vaginal itching can be caused by several things, the most common of which is a surface reaction to a chemical irritant (i.e. contact dermatitis). Some women who are severely allergic to pollens can also experience seasonal vulvar itching that corresponds to higher pollen counts. After all, the female genital area is moist and warm, much like the mucosal tissue found in the eye and nasal passages. Whether the itching is caused by an infection or topical irritation, my program for vulvar pruritus is easy and does the job:

• Avoid washing the vulva with soap, including so-called hypoallergenic varieties. The only exception is Aveeno, an oatmeal-based cleansing agent and the only true hypo-allergenic soap. Wash the affected area twice daily with Aveeno and then thoroughly rinse with soft water. Pat dry, do not rub!

• Keep the area dry. Wearing loose-fitting clothes is a *must*. Form-fitting slacks and tight jeans only aggravate the problem. Wear a dress or skirt instead. Also, panties and undergarments should be 100 percent cotton—not just cotton lined. When possible, go *al fresco* (no underwear) for periods of time to let the vulvar tissue breathe or wear nothing below the waist at night.

• Use Aveeno soap to launder your underwear. And never use fabric softener (liquid or dryer sheets), as this can cause irritation.

I've used the above program with phenomenal success in hundreds of women from youngsters to great grandmothers. Many of my patients are amazed that such a simple program succeeds when costly prescription medications have failed. If the itching persists or if redness, ulcers or lumps are present, make sure to consult your doctor. Certain types of cancer can cause itching in conjunction with the presence of a growth or ulcer.

---

### Donna's Dilemma

Donna was referred to me for persistent vaginal irritation that had not responded to over-the-counter and prescription creams and drugs. She was desperate for solutions and discouraged by the cost (ointments had cost her twenty dollars a tube) and their ineffectiveness. During our visit, Donna also told me that sex had also become painful. She likened it to having tiny cuts around the vaginal opening. Although she continued to have sex for her husband's sake, she often cringed at the prospect. (It's no wonder that so many women with these problems develop an aversion to sex.)

Donna's condition is referred to as "vulvodynia," a chronic condition that remains a mystery to much of the medical community despite the millions of dollars spent researching it. Personally, I believe it's related to some type of allergic reaction to yeast. Why? Because in severe cases, using transfer factor (orally and topically) dramatically improved the problem.

In Donna's case, I suggested vaginal acidification and a hygiene program. She came back to see me after a month. "The pain and discomfort were completely gone," she told me with a big grin. She then thanked me, but I told her that she should give herself credit for faithfully following my instructions. She's not the first woman who responded so positively to a treatment that is surprisingly simple and "unmedical."

## Nora's Dramatic Change

Nora had a history of extreme fatigue, chronic vaginal infections, severe vulvar itching, heavy menstrual periods, breast tenderness and low sex drive. She was also very prone to illness and seemed to catch every cold or sore throat that came along. She brought a large bag full of $300 worth of vaginal creams and prescription drugs with her. When I asked Nora about her dietary and exercise habits, I was not surprised to learn that her diet consisted of red meat, chicken, soda, few vegetables and no coldwater fish. Although she belonged to a health club, she got little to no exercise.

Before doing anything else, I decided to encourage Nora to change her eating habits and begin exercising. I then told her about the "dynamic duo" of genistein and natural progesterone cream and how it could help relieve her PMS and heavy periods. I also recommended that she try transfer factor to build her immune system (which was obviously failing to function properly). To top it all off, I told her about vaginal acidification and other tips that could reduce the frequency and severity of vaginal infections and itching.

When Nora came back a month later, her only complaint was some fatigue. She told me that she had followed all of my suggestions, including changing her diet and beginning an exercise program. In fact, Nora had convinced her overweight husband to start going to the gym with her. She hadn't been sick for the entire month, even though her family was plagued with colds. I smiled and asked her why she hadn't shared her transfer factor with them. Apparently she had tried, but they just didn't believe her. Thanks to the acidification program, her vaginal infections and itching were also gone. Nora chose to change her health destiny by changing her habits.

# Practical Do's and Don'ts for Preventing Infection

I tell my patients with recurring infections to keep the vaginal area cool and dry by wearing loose clothing and 100 percent cotton underwear. I also frown on the use of vaginal sprays, commercial douches and deodorants, which can alter the natural acid/alkaline balance of the vagina, predisposing it to infection. Douching is also potentially dangerous because it can force the infection up through the cervix, which could eventually cause pelvic inflammatory disease.

Research shows that women who douche on a regular basis actually develop more vaginal irritations and infections than women who don't. These women are also more prone to pelvic inflammatory disease (PID). In fact their risk is 73 percent greater. Remember that PID can lead to infertility or serious problems during pregnancy, including infections in the newborn and problems with labor and delivery. Instead of douching, choose natural treatments for yeast infections that directly target the ecosystem of the vaginal canal and boost immune defenses. (Also keep in mind that birth control pills have been associated with vaginal yeast infections.)

## Other Natural Ways to Prevent Vaginal Infections

• Avoid alcohol, white sugar and refined flour foods. The candida fungus feeds on simple sugars.

• Cut down on dairy products. Milk products may aggravate yeast infections, although low-fat yogurt with active cultures is recommended.

• Choose seafood and vegetable proteins over meat and poultry, and be careful of yeasty, moldy or fermented foods, such as aged cheeses, dried fruits or mushrooms.

## Additional Supplements to Consider

**Beneficial bacteria.** Taking 1/2 to 1 teaspoon (or two capsules) of acidophilus and bifidobacteria three times a day helps to repopulate the beneficial vaginal flora that keep candida in check.

**Transfer factor.** This supplement can help boost natural killer cells that keep fungal growth under control. Take as directed on the product label.

**Garlic.** Eat one or two raw cloves, or take garlic capsules two to three times daily. Garlic may be more effective against yeast infections than the prescription medication Nystatin.

Chapter 15

□ ▨ ▪ ▪

# Antioxidants Are Not Optional

We know a great deal more about the causes of physical disease than
we do about the causes of physical health.
– M. Scott Peck

**A question that** my patients—especially those in the baby
boomer generation—frequently ask is "How can I deal with the
complications of aging?" Whether their concerns are cosmetic
(wrinkles and age spots) or life threatening (heart disease,
Alzheimer's and other degenerative diseases), women today don't
believe life is over at fifty (or sixty or seventy, for that matter).
They want to live life to the fullest. My answer to them is always
the same—take antioxidants! True, antioxidants are not just for
women, but considering that women often live longer than men
and so are more likely to be victims of all the damage aging can
do, a supplement that slows its effects sure can't hurt!

I'm devoting an entire chapter to antioxidants because they are
absolutely critical to maintaining good health. If you do nothing
else, make sure to take a good antioxidant supplement. Why am
I so passionate about antioxidants? Because they work to neutralize the dangerous effects of certain culprit molecules you may

have heard of called free radicals. Yes, the human body produces several enzymes that neutralize free radicals. But it's hard for the body to keep up with the demand, so supplementing it with the "building blocks" of these enzymes is crucial—it enhances the body's entire defensive operation.

Antioxidant supplements have become extremely popular in recent years. Go into any health food or grocery store and you'll find countless supplements described as "the best" or "the most powerful" antioxidant. In truth, alpha lipoic acid, bromelain, coenzyme Q10, curcumin, quercitin, lutein, lycopene, beta carotene, grapeseed and pine bark extracts, and vitamins A, C and E are all good antioxidants. However, all antioxidants are not created equal, so knowing what to look for and why is what this chapter is all about.

## Modern Health Perils

Twentieth century life exposes us to a myriad of potentially harmful toxins. Every day, regardless of where or how we live, bombards us with scores of chemicals that create damaging free radicals or oxidants in our bodies. The culprits come in the form of automobile exhaust, UV rays, tobacco smoke and food additives—even the chemicals used to purify our water. Other dangerous free-radical-producing substances include:

• alcohol
• certain prescription drugs
• diagnostic and therapeutic x-rays
• gamma radiation
• herbicides
• hydrogenated and saturated fats
• pesticides
• poor diets

- rancid foods
- some of our food and water supplies
- stress
- smog
- ultraviolet light

Even exercising, as beneficial as it is, can initiate the release of free radicals. Aerobic exercise produces damaging oxidative by-products—including many that are not completely neutralized by internal safety mechanisms. As a result of constant exposure to free radicals, our risk of developing a degenerative disease increases significantly. In addition, these oxidizing agents can accelerate premature tissue breakdown causing us to age more rapidly.

## Infamous Free Radicals

A free radical is nothing more than a molecular structure containing an unpaired electron. Electrons like to coexist in pairs. These "couples" make up the chemical bond that keeps molecules from flying apart, so an unpaired electron is driven by a potent chemical force compelling it to find a mate. This molecular instinct to merge with another electron is so powerful that an unpaired molecule behaves erratically, moving about much like a weapon within cellular structures creating damage.

A free radical can destroy a protein, an enzyme or even a complete cell. To make matters worse, free radicals can multiply through a chain reaction that results in the release of thousands of dangerous cellular oxidants. In fact, it's estimated that we make a million free radicals per cell each day.

# Why Are Free Radicals So Dangerous?

Over time, unstable free radicals can cause cellular breakdown and mutation. Cells become so badly damaged that DNA codes are altered, and ultimately, immunity can be compromised. In fact, free radical damage has been associated with over sixty known diseases and disorders. Tissue breakdown from this oxidative stress can contribute to aging, arthritis, osteoporosis, heart disease and a whole host of other degenerative conditions. In some cases, cellular deterioration stimulates uncontrolled cell replication that results in cancerous tumors. Constant free radical bombardment has even been compared to being irradiated at low levels over time.

## Slowing Down the Destruction

What makes metals rust or wood decay? The presence of oxygen. It causes these materials to oxidize and break down. In short, metal oxidizes when it is exposed to air and so do we. We are basically "rusting out." Clearly, abusing our bodies makes them rust out faster, even though the effects of this abuse may not become apparent until we get older. Our bodies have an enormous ability to repair themselves, but there is a point—after years of exposure—where free radical damage becomes irreparable.

To combat oxidative damage, we need the help of antioxidant compounds. These remarkable nutrients protect us from the perils of free radicals. Antioxidants work in several ways. First of all, they actually sap energy out of a free radical and can even prevent its formation. Antioxidants are often called free radical "scavengers" because they donate electrons to free radical molecules, thereby stabilizing their structures. Simply stated, antioxidants neutralize free radicals.

## Free Radicals and High-Fat Diets

□ ▨ ■ ■

Certain dietary fats, specifically saturated and trans fats, can produce free radicals and predispose us to heart disease. Numerous research studies also support the fact that many cancers (breast cancer in particular) are diet related. Simply changing to a "low-fat" diet may not be enough. Recent studies suggest that reducing dietary fat alone may not be enough to prevent certain cancers. This may explain why some cultures that eat fatty diets, such as those in the Mediterranean, have low cancer rates. Yes, they eat a lot of fat, but the fats they eat are beneficial. By changing to a diet that includes more essential fatty acids (found in fish) and monounsaturated fats (like olive oil), you can reduce your free radical damage. Keep in mind that an excess of polyunsaturated fats like those found in corn oil and margarine can also pose a health threat. The process used to harden polyunsaturates creates the harmful acids that can contribute to cardiovascular disease.

While common-sense measures such as eating nutritiously and living a healthy lifestyle should be our first line of defense, we need extra fortification. When we take antioxidant supplements we help the body produce more of its own antioxidants (like superoxide dismutase [SOD] and glutathione peroxidase). I know what you're thinking—why not take supplements of these enzymes instead of antioxidants? Antioxidants are a better choice because the human body doesn't absorb these enzymes well. Antioxidants provide the building blocks needed to make the enzymes it needs.

Remember, taking antioxidants becomes particularly crucial if cancer or heart disease runs in your family. Moreover, any time you have surgery or are recovering from any kind of injury, free radical counts go up. Even something as simple as endometrial ablation elevates free radical levels, so I advise all of my patients who have undergone surgery to up their antioxidant intake. In my estimation, women who follow my advice recover more rapidly than those who don't.

## Show Me the Data

One of the most impressive and widely publicized research trials on antioxidants was a five-year study published in the *Journal of the National Cancer Institute.* It involved approximately thirty thousand residents of China who were given either a placebo or a dietary supplement containing one of seven vitamin-mineral combinations. Persons who received a daily dose of beta carotene, vitamin E and selenium (all antioxidants) reduced their cancer rate by 13 percent.

Moreover, the American Heart Association (AHA) recently reported that women who consumed high amounts of antioxidant-containing foods (i.e. carrots, spinach and other green vegetables) had a 33 percent lower risk of heart attack and a 71 percent lower risk of stroke than women who ate few antioxidant-containing foods. This trial involved nearly two thousand female nurses with a history of heart disease. Bottom line—the nurses who consumed the most dietary antioxidants had the greatest reduction in coronary disease.

Yet in spite of scores of studies confirming the benefits of antioxidants, the American Heart Association and the American Cancer Society continue to say that it is "premature" to recommend dietary supplements containing antioxidants. Their rational? It's not possible to say conclusively that antioxidant vitamins—as opposed to foods that are high in antioxidants—can reduce the risk of stroke or heart attack. What kind of rea-

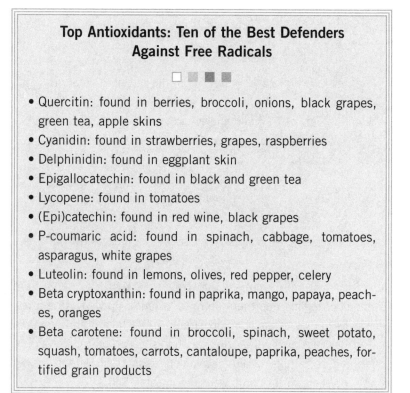

**Top Antioxidants: Ten of the Best Defenders Against Free Radicals**

- Quercitin: found in berries, broccoli, onions, black grapes, green tea, apple skins
- Cyanidin: found in strawberries, grapes, raspberries
- Delphinidin: found in eggplant skin
- Epigallocatechin: found in black and green tea
- Lycopene: found in tomatoes
- (Epi)catechin: found in red wine, black grapes
- P-coumaric acid: found in spinach, cabbage, tomatoes, asparagus, white grapes
- Luteolin: found in lemons, olives, red pepper, celery
- Beta cryptoxanthin: found in paprika, mango, papaya, peaches, oranges
- Beta carotene: found in broccoli, spinach, sweet potato, squash, tomatoes, carrots, cantaloupe, paprika, peaches, fortified grain products

soning is this? It should a "no brainer." The official stance on the validity of taking antioxidants defies all reason. Yes, eating foods high in antioxidants is a best-case scenario. Unfortunately, the majority of Americans aren't doing it. Supplementation is the next best thing.

## Antioxidants: The Missing Link

Laura came to see me because she was suffering from chronic fatigue, chest pain and insomnia. Although she was already using my diet and exercise program, her health wasn't optimal. After a thorough exam, I suggested that she add an antioxidant mix of

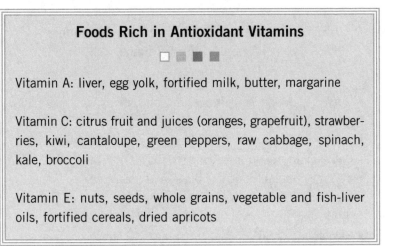

**Foods Rich in Antioxidant Vitamins**

Vitamin A: liver, egg yolk, fortified milk, butter, margarine

Vitamin C: citrus fruit and juices (oranges, grapefruit), strawberries, kiwi, cantaloupe, green peppers, raw cabbage, spinach, kale, broccoli

Vitamin E: nuts, seeds, whole grains, vegetable and fish-liver oils, fortified cereals, dried apricots

quercitin, curcumin, lycopene and grapeseed extract to her current supplement regime and then return for a follow-up visit. After a few weeks, Laura saw a rapid improvement in her health and stamina. During her last visit, she told me that she couldn't believe that something so simple could have such a dramatic effect on her health. For her, antioxidants were the missing link.

## Foods with Antioxidant Clout

Taking an antioxidant supplement shouldn't be substituted for a diet high in antioxidant-rich foods. The following is a list of antioxidant "heavyweights" as rated by the *Journal of Agricultural and Food Chemistry:*

| Food | Antioxidant Capacity |
| --- | --- |
| Garlic | 19.4 |
| Kale | 17.7 |
| Strawberries | 15.6 |
| Spinach | 12.6 |

| | |
|---|---|
| Brussels sprouts | 9.8 |
| Plums | 9.49 |
| Broccoli | 8.9 |
| Beets | 8.4 |
| Red Bell Pepper | 7.1 |
| Oranges | 7.5 |
| Grapes | 7.39 |
| Kiwi | 6.02 |
| Pink Grapefruit | 4.83 |
| Onion | 4.5 |
| Corn | 4.0 |
| Eggplant | 3.9 |
| Cauliflower | 3.8 |
| Potato | 3.1 |
| Cabbage | 3.0 |
| Leaf lettuce | 2.6 |
| Banana | 2.21 |
| Apple | 2.18 |
| Carrot | 2.1 |
| String bean | 2.0 |
| Yellow squash | 2.1 |
| Tomato | 1.89 |
| Pear | 1.37 |
| Melon | 0.97 |
| Celery | 0.6 |
| Cucumber | 0.5 |

With legions of baby boomers currently cresting "over the hill," anti-aging compounds have a ready-made market. Jonathan Swift once said that everyone desires to live long, but no one wants to be old. While there is no fountain of youth, disease and aging don't have to go hand-in-hand. Granted, we can't stop the formation of free radicals in the body, but we can modify their potentially disastrous effects by eating smart, not smoking, and taking a "kick-butt" antioxidant supplement every day. If you start now and stay diligent, don't be surprised when family and friends ask you how you manage to stay so young.

Chapter 16

□ ▦ ■ ■

# Transfer Factor:
# The Immune Connection

Transfer factors are small proteins that "transfer" the ability to express cell-mediated immunity from immune donors to nonimmune recipients.
— *Molecular Medicine*, 6 April, 2000

**It's not a** vitamin, mineral, herb or hormone. But it may be the most promising discovery in immunology and preventive medicine to date. You may be wondering why I would devote a whole chapter to a supplement that boosts immune function. It is true that transfer factor is not a woman's supplement per se, but after using it for over eight years, I am convinced that what it offers women (and men) is too valuable to be ignored. In fact, the merits of using transfer factor could fill another book. I believe that transfer factor (TF) should be a key part of anyone's prescription for maximum health and disease prevention.

After my fight with cancer, I realized that conventional medicine had very little to offer in the way of protection. Make no mistake, once cancer appears in one part of your body, your risk of getting it somewhere else goes up. Both my father and mother died of cancer; my son has had a melanoma; my oldest daughter had a pre-melanotic lesion on her ear; my mother-in-law had breast cancer, and my wife's sister had breast cancer twice before she died of a massive stroke. Obviously we were doing a lousy job of preventing cancer in our family. So I began to look elsewhere for answers.

Eventually I crossed paths with a naturopathic physician who told me about a natural product that not only boosted immune function, but also calmed an overactive immune system—often seen in people with autoimmune diseases (and something my youngest daughter struggled with). What was this miracle supplement? It was called transfer factor (TF). My initial skepticism turned to intense interest, so I reviewed all and any available literature on transfer factor. Here was a scientifically supported compound purported to successfully work with the body's own immune system, not in spite of it (as is the case with conventional treatments like antibiotics and chemo). If these claims were true, I thought, transfer factor could revolutionize the practice of medicine.

## My Experience with Transfer Factor

I have used transfer factor for years now, and have found that my resistance to disease has dramatically improved. I rarely get the flu or a cold anymore, and when I encounter someone who does, I always ask them, "Why are you sick? You know, you don't have to be."

I advise all of my patients to take transfer factor. To date, I have put over one thousand women on TF. I have to laugh (but I'm not surprised) when husbands of my patients ask to try it. The conversion usually comes after a battle with the flu, during which their wives remain perfectly healthy! Cancer patients in particular can benefit from transfer factor because many cancer treatments are detrimental to the immune system. More than one woman who has sailed through chemo after using transfer factor has asked me, "What's in this stuff?" As I said, I have been taking TF daily for more than eight years, and my immune system is stronger than ever. (In fact, transfer factor is the only thing that helped me get rid of persistent canker sores that have plagued me since I was a child.)

## You Can Lead a Horse to Water . . .

At this point you may be asking yourself, if transfer factor is so important, why haven't I heard of it? Your doctor probably isn't telling you about transfer factor for the same reasons he doesn't recommend genistein or progesterone cream—he isn't familiar with them or he doesn't believe in the validity of complementary medicine.

When I tell my medical colleagues about my experiences with transfer factor and the mountains of research supporting its use, they don't openly rebuke me. Of course, these are the same doctors who came to me to learn several of my new gynecological procedures (cryosurgery, colposcopy, endometrial ablation, etc.). In spite of their polite responses (and to my disappointment), none of these physicians use transfer factor for themselves or their patients. I believe their predictable response to TF was a knee-jerk reaction of the worst kind.

## What Exactly Is Transfer Factor?

More than fifty years ago, scientists isolated tiny immune molecules made up of amino acids that relay immune messages between immune cells. Called transfer factors, these messengers are able to educate cells about present and potential dangers from bacteria, viruses, parasites and other microbes. Basically, transfer factors help the immune system recognize and respond to infections and other threats your body is exposed to every day.

Transfer factor is abundantly found in the colostrum of breast milk. When a mother nurses her baby, transfer factors from her more experienced immune system pass to her baby via the colostrum. These immune "tutors" give the newborn's immature immune system the advantages of the mother's more experienced one. This transfer of immune information protects the baby until its immune system can make transfer factor on its own.

## Transfer Factor Is Sophisticated Immune Support

Our immune system's ability to accurately recognize foreign intruders and separate them from the body's own healthy cells determines our survival. Our immune cells must be able to sort through trillions of cells and identify friends from foe. Microbes, toxins and even cancer cells that are not recognized and disposed of pose a serious risk. It is estimated that the immune system has the ability to react to over 100 million different antigens (codes on cells that identify them). Keep in mind, however, that it may still lack information on tens of thousands of antigens. Without this immunity data, the body is more vulnerable to attack.

This is where the real benefit of transfer factor comes in. It helps fill the gaps by educating cells about antigens they have never encountered. Transfer factor can also coordinate, activate and suppress immune cells according to need as well as improve cell-to-cell communication. As a result, the immune system is better able to identify a threat, respond to it and remember it, should it encounter the threat again. This makes for stronger and more efficient immune function, and all without any side effects.

And because transfer factor proteins are not species specific, those produced by a cow can work just as effectively in humans.

This means that transfer factos extracted from cow colostrum (through a special, patented process) can be concentrated and offered in supplement form to humans. The ability to transfer immune data has the potential to revolutionize the way we look at disease prevention.

## TF and the Yeast Wars

Vickie was a thirty-eight-year-old patient who had been using antibiotics for recurrent bladder and severe vaginal yeast infections. I suggested that she stop using antibiotics and begin a course of transfer factor and acidification (discussed in Chapter 14). Her response to the treatment was dramatic. When I saw her three months later, she said that this was the first time in years that she had been free of infection. More importantly, she had not taken any antibiotics for three months. I suggested that she come back to see me in six months to check on her progress. Four months passed without further infections, so she stopped taking TF, thinking that she was "well."

Soon after she stopped taking transfer factor, Vickie developed sinusitis and was given an antibiotic by her primary physician. Within a few days, she developed a yeast infection and within the month, she suffered another bladder infection. Since then, Vickie hasn't failed to take TF and has been free of bladder, sinus and vaginal yeast infections for over three years.

# The Three-Fold Benefits of TF

When you take transfer factor, you will experience these three benefits:

1. Your immune system is strengthened so that when new viruses or bacteria invade your body, your heightened immune cells

react more rapidly. By so doing, the immune system prevents the foreign organism from getting a toehold; consequently, even if you do get sick, the infection will be milder. In fact, a 1996 issue of *Biotherapy* reported that transfer factors can stimulate an immune system response in less than twenty-four hours.

2. When you take transfer factor, you store these borrowed messenger molecules in your own immune data banks. As a result, when you are invaded by an organism that these molecules are already familiar with, your immune system is able to recognize the invader quickly and initiate an attack specific to that particular microorganism—even without prior exposure to it.

3. If you have an overactive immune system (common in autoimmune diseases like arthritis, lupus, and multiple sclerosis), transfer factors can suppress immune responses that inadvertently attack healthy tissue. Normalized immune function ultimately means better health.

## Transfer Factor: From My Personal Notes

My fifteen-year-old daughter was diagnosed with juvenile arthritis when she was eleven after suffering with swollen and extremely tender joints. This had been going on for some time before she brought it to my attention. When I examined her joints, my heart sank. I knew immediately that it was arthritis.

My wife promptly took her to our pediatrician, who confirmed the diagnosis and referred her to a pediatric rheumatologist at the University of Utah specializing in childhood arthritis. (There are fewer than fifty such specialists in the United States.) He suggested we give our daughter a very powerful anti-inflammatory drug. The side effects of this drug are extensive in adults, so I couldn't help but wonder what it would do to an eleven-year-old girl.

I consulted with another pediatrician who had been using transfer factor in his patients. He suggested that we give her six capsules a day plus a capsule of a special joint medication manufactured by the same company. Within six weeks, our daughter was pain-free, and her swelling had dramatically decreased.

Well, she's a teenager now and isn't nearly as diligent about taking the immune-modifying supplement plan we designed for her years ago. She still experiences a little swelling and an occasional twinge of pain in her thumbs, and once in a while, her knee joints will swell after vigorous exercise. Still, the improvement is remarkable, and more importantly, she did it without harsh drug therapy. She is an avid snowboarder and plans to try out for the lacrosse team next spring. You have no idea how thankful my wife and I are for transfer factor. The results continue to be nothing short of spectacular.

## TF Is Backed by Sound Scientific Data

To date, over three thousand well-documented clinical studies and papers have been published on transfer factors and their immune benefits, at an estimated cost of $40 million over the last fifty years. Scores of well-respected, international scientists and physicians have established the effectiveness and safety of transfer factors in boosting immune function. TF has emerged as a "heavyweight" in health maintenance worldwide.

Recently, a symposium on transfer factors was held in Italy where TF researcher Dr. D. Viza spoke about the potential of transfer factor in an era when "the toll of several diseases, such as cancer, continues to rise and the pathogenesis of AIDS remains elusive." The following are just a small sampling of possible applications for transfer factor:

• Clinical studies in Japan and China have been able to prevent the immunosuppressive effects of chemotherapy by using transfer factor isolates.

## The Chicken and the Egg

□ ▨ ▇ ▨

Studies are currently underway to extract transfer factor from chicken eggs. That's right—eggs. As I mentioned earlier, all kinds of animals make transfer factors. By using extremely sophisticated methodology, scientists have been able to make "designer" transfer factor molecules in chicken eggs that target specific organisms. These products are now undergoing testing to determine what role they might have in medicine. Imagine a transfer factor molecule that works specifically against the AIDS, West Nile or recently emerging SARS virus. The possibilities are endless, but more testing is required before they can be made available to the public.

• A study by a pediatrician in Maine found that eighty-eight children who used TF daily experienced a 74 percent reduction in reported illness and an 84 percent reduction in antibiotic use. Moreover, the children experienced no side effects from daily use.

• Researchers in Japan found that transfer factor supplementation was successful for children with juvenile rheumatoid arthritis who were unresponsive to steroids and immunosupressants.

• A February 1999 study in the *Journal of the American Nutraceutical Association* published a review of nearly two hundred products believed to enhance the action of natural killer (NK) cells (immune cells that seek out and destroy foreign invaders). Among those found to be most successful were shiitake mushroom (with a 42 percent enhancement) and echinacea (with 43 percent). However, a test of transfer factor produced an amazing 103 percent enhancement of NK activity.

## A Man in Montana

I came to know a man named Jim in Bozeman, Montana. He had multiple myeloma, a very serious and potentially fatal cancer, and was so incapacitated by the illness, he could barely walk. I gave him transfer factor (combined with a variety of other immune-enhancing compounds), and after a short time, he experienced a remarkable remission. Last I heard, Jim was climbing a local Montana mountain. Though his cancer may return, the extraordinary effects of his immune-boosting protocol cannot be underestimated, or worse yet, ignored.

## "I Had Forgotten How It Felt to Be Healthy"

Marilyn was perimenopausal and what I like to call "immune challenged" when she came to see me. I realized that we had to build her immunity before addressing her gynecological problems. She was catching every virus that came along and was sick and tired of being sick and tired. I realized immediately that Marilyn also was stressed to the max—a factor that can wear down resistance to disease.

---

### Possible Uses for Transfer Factor

| | |
|---|---|
| allergies | hives |
| asthma | infections |
| cancer | lupus |
| chronic fatigue | multiple sclerosis |
| Crohn's disease | psoriasis |
| cold and flu | rheumatoid arthritis |
| eczema | sinusitis |
| fibromyalgia | tuberculosis |
| hepatitis B/C | type I diabetes |

I told Marilyn that she needed to manage her stress. She started a yoga class, got regular massage treatments and went to bed earlier. She also drastically reduced her intake of red meat, sugar and white flour, started an exercise program and started taking transfer factor daily. When I saw her for a follow-up exam, she was a different person. "I had forgotten how it felt to be healthy," she told me. "I can't believe more doctors don't recommend lifestyle changes and transfer factor to their patients."

## The Last Word on TF

Transfer factor is nothing less than an amazing natural compound that should be used by people of all ages. Last year alone, I flew over two hundred thousand miles throughout the United States and Europe, and I never became ill. We all know about the microbial hazards of recirculated plane cabin air, and yet here I sit, infection free. Let me reiterate at this point that I would not presume to recommend any natural product unless it came with impressive scientific credentials. Like genistein, TF had to win me over. Naturally, when word got out that I was interested in natural treatments, a number of prominent companies approached me with their line of products. Unfortunately, the science supporting many of their flagship supplements was lacking. Consequently, so was my interest. Transfer factor, on the other hand, withstood my intense scrutiny and proved its worth.

In a time when bacteria and viruses are mutating, causing new and potentially fatal diseases resistant to anything currently available in our arsenal of medicines, superior immune competency is crucial. We've already seen what Legionnaire's disease and West Nile virus can do. Now we face a new viral threat called severe acute respiratory syndrome (SARS), which has recently surfaced in Asia, North America and Europe. As of this writing, hundreds of SARS cases had been reported in the United States and Canada (as well as numerous Asian countries), and the death toll from the infection continues to mount. So what does that mean for all of us? While scientists scramble to find a cure for this new and insidious virus, we need to fortify our own immune defenses with compounds like transfer factor.

Chapter 17

□ ▨ ▣ ▨

# For Men Only

*The man who questions opinions is wise—the man who*
*argues with facts is a fool.*
*— Unknown*

**Although I specialize** in women's health care, I know that what's
good for the goose is also good for the gander, so I want to take a
minute to talk directly to men (wives and girlfriends, if you are
reading, take note). As you probably know, men are vulnerable to
many of the same diseases that afflict women—and often for the
same reasons. Heart disease is the number one killer of both
sexes. Infertility, sexual dysfunction and cancer also plague men
and women.

Many of these health problems are preventable (to some
degree or another). Although men often have access to better
health care than women, they are less likely to get regular medical
checkups. I know because I've been guilty of this myself—and as
a doctor, I should know better. Ignoring my health nearly cost me
my life. Without the insistence of my wife to get a suspicious
mole checked out, I probably wouldn't be here today.

I know I am not the only man that has ever had a blasé attitude about his health. I was chatting with a top executive with a major Wall Street firm on a recent cross-country flight. This man was in his early fifties and looked trim and healthy, so I was surprised to learn that five years earlier he had a "coronary episode." He told me that five metal stints now kept his arteries working (at a price tag of nearly $40,000!), and he would need another stint replacement in a few years. Despite the seriousness of his condition, he confided to me that he still regularly enjoyed thick, juicy steak dinners. After all, the stints seemed to be working, he pointed out. I retorted point-blank that I didn't know what his doctor had told him, but if he didn't make any lifestyle changes, he probably wouldn't live much past sixty. In essence this man was willing to "spend" years of his life in order to eat anything he wanted. I must have made my point, because follow-up phone calls revealed that he had changed to eating salmon instead of beef.

Make no mistake, guys. Having a cavalier attitude about your health can result in premature death. As I have already told the ladies, the best way to protect yourself from heart disease, cancer, diabetes and countless other diseases, is to eat a healthier diet (soy isn't just for women), exercise regularly (your monthly basketball game isn't enough), take a few essential supplements and form a better relationship with your doctor. But to create a working partnership with a physician, you have to be willing to see one, even if you feel perfectly fine. It's called a physical exam, and you shouldn't wait until you're in the middle of a health crisis to get one.

## Making a Checkup Count

Not all physical exams are created equal. In fact, routine physical exams given to heads of corporations and those done for insurance purposes can be a bit of a sham. My own father, who was a high-level executive, had an in-house physical every six months. Yet without warning, he went into serious heart failure when he was fifty-five. Although my father had showed evidence of cardiovascular disease, his doctor failed to diagnose his condition during earlier periodic exams. Even after the problem was found, his doctor never encouraged him to change his diet. He was given prescriptions for digitalis and high blood pressure medication and that was that.

Later, at the age of sixty-one, my father learned that he had an incurable form of kidney cancer. Prior to this diagnosis, his doctors ignored the fair amount of protein that kept showing up in his urine—a sign that something was wrong—and sadly, he died of the disease. I have no doubt that my father's cancer was the result of the petrochemicals he was exposed to while working in oil fields years before. I also know that a good doctor would have discovered the cancer when he first developed high blood pressure (his hypertension was caused by the kidney disease)—something that might have saved his life.

My father-in-law's acute gallbladder disease also slipped by his doctor. Of course, doctors aren't infallible. I'm not trying to be overly critical of my colleagues, but I do believe that as members of the medical profession, we need to be vigilant. When symptoms appear, we need to take every action necessary to figure out what's wrong and how to fix it. And at the risk of sounding repetitive, we need to—whenever possible—take steps to keep our patients healthy, not to merely step in to repair the damage.

## Change Your Lifestyle

Men, the same advice applies to you. Don't wait for a health crisis to make vital lifestyle changes. When something is wrong, get it checked out immediately instead of hoping it goes away. If you take an active role in staying healthy, you have a distinct advantage over the thousands of men who lead stressful lives, eat lousy diets, get little or no exercise and rarely seek medical advice.

Scores of studies tell us that we can reverse heart disease, prevent diabetes and improve our sexual health if we make a few lifestyle changes. For example, according to an August 2000 study in *Urology*, regular exercise (that spends about 200 calories per day) significantly lowers a man's risk for erectile dysfunction (ED), even if the man does not begin exercising until midlife. Burning more than 200 calories a day lowered that risk even more. The men in the study were followed for almost ten years, and they had no subsequent problems with impotence. A 2002 article in *European Journal of Cancer Prevention* lists monounsaturated oils (such as olive oil), fish and fish oils, fiber, and fruits and vegetables as proven heart protectors that reduce cancer risk. Culprits such as saturated fats, fried foods, smoking, and excessive salt intake are listed as factors that raise your risk of cancer and heart disease. Obviously diet and exercise play a larger role in our health than many of us believe. Now is the time to take action.

## Cardiac Recovery: Have Your Cake and Eat It Too?

Jim was a seventy-year-old man who had experienced a series of massive heart attacks. He underwent the customary cardiac surgery, and when I saw him, his attitude—like so many other men—was "why bother to live healthier when I can just pop a pill?" Eventually, I convinced him to try my suggestions. He quit smoking, started taking a good multivitamin and mineral supplement (as well as genistein and transfer factor), changed his diet, and began exercising. After a few weeks, he got better—a lot better. He went from a man who could barely shuffle across the room, to one who walked three miles a day. Show me a pill that can do that.

But this story doesn't have a happy ending. Unfortunately, in the midst of all this progress, Jim's doctor put him on a cholesterol-lowering drug that gave his stomach fits. His gastrointestinal problems caused him to stop exercising, and he eventually slipped back into his old ways—smoking, eating red meat, and so on. Let me emphasize here that all the drugs in the world won't confer the kind of health Jim could have enjoyed with lifestyle changes.

# What Healthy Men Do

Since I made positive changes in my lifestyle several years ago, my health has greatly improved. I am energetically entering my "Medicare years," cancer free and healthier than ever, despite a grim family (and personal) history of health conditions.

I recently met an eighty-seven-year-old neurologist—still practicing—who had just started an organization to address the issue of transitory amnesia. I have to tell you, this guy is sharp and in excellent physical condition—he still plays tennis four times a week. When I asked him his secret to his vitality, he smiled and said, "Health and long life really boil down to diet. I don't eat much meat, I eat plenty of fruits and vegetables, and I'm a great believer in portion control. We've got a real problem in this country—the American diet is a complete train wreck."

With all that medical science knows about health and disease, this doctor's story should be the norm, not the exception. Unfortunately, many men live out their "golden years" (if they live that long) suffering from heart disease, impotence, prostate disorders, digestive problems, and diabetes. If you're interested in changing your health destiny, I have included below a number of habits every healthy man should adopt:

## 1. Healthy men watch their meat and fat intake

I know, I know, men love to barbecue. Nothing tastes quite as good as a smoked prime rib or mesquite grilled T-bone steak.

Unfortunately, that steak you're throwing on the grill is full of saturated fats, not to mention possible hormones, steroids and antibiotics. Beef also contains arachidonic acid, which promotes prostate cancer in animals. In one study, men who consumed a high amount saturated fat (from meat and dairy) for over five years had over three times the risk of dying from prostate cancer compared with men consuming the least amount of saturated fat. To make matters worse, saturated fat raises cholesterol levels. The American Heart Association recommends that everyone should keep their intake of saturated fat between 7 and 10 percent of their total daily calories.

That's why you won't find any beef at my house. I advise men to choose salmon instead. Men who regularly consume fatty fish such as salmon and mackerel are up to three times less likely to develop prostate cancer over a thirty-year period than men who don't. Coldwater fish contain omega-3 fatty acids (as do pumpkin and flax seeds), which have been shown to inhibit the growth of prostate cancer cells. Omega-3s also can lower "bad" (LDL) cholesterol, help blood sugar regulation, lower stroke risk, and promote heart health. The American Heart Association suggests replacing saturated fat with omega-3 fats and monounsaturated fats (found in olive oil, avocados and some nuts).

If you just can't live without your red meat, then spend a little more for range-fed varieties (deer, elk, buffalo and specialty beef). Range-fed meat is leaner (often less than 10 percent saturated fat) and contains more omega-3 fatty acids. But remember, even range-fed meat should be eaten infrequently and in small portions.

Although poultry may seem like a good alternative to beef, it's certainly not perfect. I try to choose free-range, organic poultry and eggs gathered from free-range chickens. Eggs from free-range chickens also contain more omega-3s. Also, skinless white meat is preferable over dark meat since it has less fat.

Decrease your intake of dairy products as well. Data from a

long-term study suggests that eating dairy products like milk, cheese and ice cream can raise your risk of prostate cancer. Scientists at the Harvard School of Public Health tracked 20,885 men for eleven years, and more than a thousand of them developed prostate cancer. From their research, scientists concluded that men who consumed dairy products were more likely to develop the disease.

Lastly, men should monitor their intake of trans fats, found in margarine, baked goods (packaged) and restaurant fried foods. Some studies suggest that these fats are more dangerous than saturated fat when it comes to heart disease. Trans fats impair blood vessel function (a risk factor for heart disease and diabetes), raise bad (LDL) cholesterol levels and decrease good (HDL) cholesterol. Consequently, the American Heart Association recommends that we avoid margarines, shortening, french fries, doughnuts, cookies, crackers and other processed or fried foods that contain hydrogenated fats.

## 2. Healthy men eat plenty of fruits and vegetables

Besides providing the body with necessary nutrients for health and longevity, eating a variety of fruits and vegetables has been shown to substantially lower cancer risk. Researchers have found that men who eat twenty-eight or more servings of vegetables per week have a 35 percent lower risk of prostate cancer compared with men who eat fewer than fourteen servings per week. And men who eat three or more servings of cruciferous vegetables (such as cauliflower and broccoli) per week have a 41 percent less chance of prostate cancer compared with men who eat less than one serving per week. Cruciferous vegetables contain isothiocyanates, which activate enzymes that neutralize carcinogens (and which are the same compounds that protect women from breast cancer).

### 3. Healthy men know soy isn't just for women

The genistein found in soy foods such as tofu, soy milk and some soy protein powders aren't just good for women—they provide men hormonal protection as well. And its heart benefits are too good to pass up. In fact, according to a study in the *New England Journal of Medicine,* replacing animal protein with soy protein reduced LDL cholesterol levels (the "bad" kind), without interfering with levels of HDL cholesterol (the "good" kind). Consequently, the FDA has approved health claims on product labels associating soy protein with a reduced risk for heart disease.

Soy also helps to inhibit the growth of prostate cancer cells and even works to destroy them. A study out of the University of Alabama found that soy inhibits protein kinase, which can contribute to abnormal cell replication. It also blocks the action of bad testosterone in the prostate gland much in the same way that it protects breast tissue against estrogen exposure. Bad testosterone causes changes in prostate tissue that can lead to the formation of cancer.

A Finnish study found that animals given a soybean feed consisting of 7 percent roasted soybean meal, showed a significantly lower incidence of prostate tissue abnormalities when artificially stimulated with hormones. Another study showed that test rats given cancerous tissue that ate a diet consisting of 33 percent defatted soy flour developed smaller tumors than control rats on a soy-free diet. In fact, Harvard researchers are currently looking at soy isoflavones as a treatment for prostate cancer.

A man's risk for colon cancer is also reduced with soy consumption. A 1996 study in the *American Journal of Epidemiology* found that eating at least one serving of soy per week could cut a person's risk for developing polyps in the colon (a precursor for colon cancer) by 50 percent. Other studies suggest that soy lowers colorectal cancer risk. If you can't get used to eating soy foods, then take a genistein supplement every day.

## 4. Healthy men take supplements

I have heard women complain over and over again that getting their husbands to take vitamins is almost impossible. Come on guys! What's so hard about popping a few pills with breakfast? There's nothing to it. Take a good vitamin and mineral supplement combined with a strong antioxidant blend that has extra selenium. A crossover study of thousands of men showed that selenium (a trace mineral) reduced the risk of prostate, lung and colon cancer by a whopping fifty percent. And in a double-blind study of mostly nonsmoking men, supplementation with beta-carotene led to a 32 percent reduction in risk of prostate cancer in men who were low in the nutrient. Still not convinced? Read more about the importance of vitamin and mineral supplements in Chapter 6.

## 5. Healthy men exercise regularly

Regular physical activity can prevent obesity, diabetes, depression, cardiovascular disease and many other conditions. It also boosts endurance and stamina, increases circulation to the brain, expedites the removal of toxins from the lymphatic system and improves digestion. With all these advantages, why don't doctors push their patients to exercise? Regardless, the responsibility is ultimately yours. If you make the commitment to get physically fit, tell your doctor what you need, and expect his or her support!

Men should aim for at least thirty minutes of cardiovascular activity three to six days a week. Walking, jogging, cycling, swimming, stair climbing and the treadmill or Nordic Track are all good aerobic activities. Be sure to incorporate warm-up and cool-down segments into your cardiovascular routine to decrease your chance of injury. It's also important to include three thirty-minute sessions of resistance training each week. Weightlifting, resistance cords and weight machines found at gyms are good choices. Exercise is also the best way to get rid of that gut. Your risk of colon cancer doubles if your waist size exceeds forty inches. Finally, remember to stretch after each exercise session. Building flexibility will help you avoid injury.

## Preventing Prostate Cancer

More than two hundred thousand new cases of prostate cancer are diagnosed every year, and 31,000 men die from the disease annually, making it the most common form of cancer in men. Even though more than 75 percent of prostate cancer cases are diagnosed in men over the age of sixty-five, prostate cancer doesn't have to be a consequence of aging, and scientists have not identified a gene responsible for the disease. Although men with a family history of prostate cancer have a higher risk of developing the disease, heredity accounts for less than 10 percent of all cases.

So how do we explain why so many men get prostate cancer? It's simple—poor diet, inactivity and obesity play a major role. There are more than enough studies confirming the notion that staying at a healthy weight and consuming more vegetables and less animal products can prevent the development of prostate cancer. Whether men want to face it or not, I believe it all starts with their diets.

Prostate cancer rates in America are almost ten times higher than those in Japan. Yet Japanese men who settle here and adopt typical American eating habits lose that advantage. The standard Asian diet is full of vegetables, legumes, soy and fish, and includes minimal amounts of red meat. Japanese men get around 40 to 70 mg of genistein from their meals compared to American men, who typically consume less than 1 mg. According to one study, men who consume 200 mg of soy milk a day are reported to have a significantly lower risk of prostate cancer compared with other men. I've been taking genistein in supplement form for over seven years. With a father who died from kidney cancer and a brother who has had prostate problems, I want all the protection I can get.

Treating prostate cancer is often problematic. It also has a high rate of recurrence. Even if a man is not treated with radiation and chemotherapy, other treatments, such as androgen deprivation therapy (ADT), can have serious side effects. A March 2002 study in the *Journal of the National Cancer Institute* found that 80 percent of men treated with this therapy became impotent (compared with 30 percent who did not receive treatment). Other side effects included breast swelling and hot flashes, and researchers determined that these men actually had a higher risk of their cancer progressing than men not using ADT. Some men prefer a "watch-and-wait" approach, foregoing all treatment until they see whether the cancer progresses. None of these options sound very good to me.

Luckily, there are ways to reduce your chances of prostate cancer. First, give up a sedentary lifestyle. Inactivity and excess body weight increase cancer risk. In addition, it's important to begin screening for cancer at fifty if you have no risk factors for the disease and at forty if you do. Switching to a diet low in fat, meat and dairy is also important. The American Cancer Society recommends replacing high-fat foods with fruits, vegetables and whole grains. I also recommend eating soy foods regularly or taking a soy supplement daily, as well as increasing your antioxidant intake. Antioxidants like vitamin E and lycopene (found in tomatoes and tomato products) may decrease your prostate cancer risk by scavenging for cancer-causing free radicals. Below is a complete list of supplements for prostate health.

# Key Supplements for Prostate Health

*Vitamin E:* According to a recent Finnish study, vitamin E supplementation protects against prostate cancer. The incidence of prostate cancer and the death rate from the disease were significantly lower among male smokers who took vitamin E supplements than those who did not. In addition, the incidence of prostate cancer was 32 percent lower among men who took vitamin E (alone or with beta carotene) than among those who did not, and the death rate from the disease was 41 percent lower among men who took vitamin E. Researchers concluded that long-term daily supplementation with 50 mg (75 I.U.) of vitamin E was associated with a substantial reduction in incidence and mortality of prostate cancer.

*Selenium:* This mineral has several anticancer actions. Interestingly, low soil levels of selenium have been associated with increased prostate cancer incidence. In one study, over nine hundred men received 200 mcg of selenium or a placebo daily for over four years. Then they were followed for an additional six-and-a-half years. For those men who initially had normal PSA (prostate-specific antigen) levels, selenium supplementation was responsible for a 63 percent reduction in their incidence of prostate cancer. And in another study, over four thousand men—followed for four years—benefited from selenium supplementation. The men received either 200 mcg of selenium or a placebo, and because there was such a dramatic decrease in the frequency of new cancer (prostate, colon and lung) in men taking the supplement, the study stopped early for ethical reasons. It just wouldn't be right to continue to give men a placebo when selenium had such a protective impact against cancer.

*Zinc:* Zinc levels can be low in men with prostate cancer. In some studies zinc supplementation actually interfered with the growth of prostate cancer cells. The prostate gland stores zinc, which means that much higher concentrations of the mineral exist in the prostate gland than in other locations. Zinc also impacts the activity of the 5 alpha-reductase enzyme, that affects the rate in which testosterone converts to dihydrotestosterone or DHT (the "bad" kind). Zinc is also vital for proper immune function.

*Vitamin B6:* This vitamin enhances zinc absorption and its chemical conversion in the prostate. Data from the Second National Health and Nutrition Examination Survey (NHANES II) reported that 71 percent of males consume less than the RDA for vitamin B6 on a daily basis. B vitamins are also vital for the maintenance of the immune defenses that protect us against the growth of malignant tumors in the body.

*Saw Palmetto:* A new study published in a recent issue of *Urology* examined the effects of saw palmetto (160 mg taken twice daily) in eighty-five men over the course of six months. Men taking the herb reported a greater improvement in prostate symptoms compared to those taking a placebo. Over the last decade, double-blind clinical trials have proven that 320 mg per day of the liposterolic extract of saw palmetto berries is a safe and effective treatment for the symptoms of BPH, (benign prostatic hyperplasia). A recent review of studies published in the *Journal of the American Medical Association* concluded that saw palmetto extract was as effective as finasteride (Proscar) for the treatment of BPH. The clinical effectiveness of saw palmetto has been shown in trials lasting six months to three years.

*Pygeum:* This extract has been approved in Germany, France and Italy as a remedy for benign prostatic hypertrophy. Controlled studies published over the past twenty-five years show that pygeum is safe and effective for men with BPH of mild or moderate severity. These studies used 50 to 100 mg of pygeum extract (standardized to contain 13 percent total sterols) twice per day. The triterpenoids found in this botanical help to promote urination; its phytosterols fight inflammation, and its ferulic esters help expedite the removal of cholesterol deposits that accompany BPH.

*Lycopene:* Abundantly found in tomatoes, this compound provides specific protection against prostate cancer. Multiple studies have linked a tomato-rich diet to reduced prostate cancer risk, and now researchers have isolated lycopene, an antioxidant, as the reason behind this effect. In a study of over 47,000 men, researchers found that frequent tomato/lycopene intake was associated with a reduced risk for prostate cancer. A great way to make sure you get enough lycopene is to consume a tablespoon of concentrated tomato paste daily.

## Male Infertility Issues

According to the Center for Male Reproductive Medicine, more than 15 percent of couples have trouble conceiving a child after more than a year of trying, and male infertility plays a role in nearly half of those cases. About one in twenty-five men are believed to suffer from fertility problems. The top causes of male infertility include a low sperm count, abnormal sperm shape or size, slow sperm movement or motility, and problems with the semen. Genes, physiology and lifestyle also play a role.

Certain antibiotics, radiation and chemotherapy, testosterone deficiencies, fevers or untreated infections (including STDs), and excessive amounts of stress may inhibit fertility. Other factors for male infertility include smoking, illicit drug use, heavy drinking, being overweight or underweight, nutrient deficiencies and exposure to environmental (or occupational) toxins. I recently ran across a newspaper article that linked falling sperm counts in Britain and other industrialized nations to pollution. According to various studies, the average sperm count has dropped by more than half over the past fifty years—from about 160 million sperm per milliliter of semen to 66 million. In other words, the typical male now produces only about a third as much sperm as a hamster. Culprit chemicals include DDT and other pesticides,

PCBs, phthalates, artificial estrogens, etc. Many of these chemicals are hormone disruptors that negatively impact both male and female fertility.

## Treating Infertility

There are many treatments available to men with fertility problems, but many of these treatments are complicated and may not be covered by insurance. I advise all couples who have been trying unsuccessfully to conceive for over a year to talk to their doctor and get tested. I also suggest that they try lifestyle changes before undergoing any serious or expensive procedures. This is especially true for young couples, since about half of all couples who fail to conceive in the first year will go on to conceive naturally in the second year. Of course for some men, congenital defects, structural abnormalities of the reproductive organs, sperm antibodies, or in-utero DES exposure may also play a role. For them, lifestyle changes will not correct infertility (but a healthy lifestyle sure can't hurt).

To promote fertility, do the following:

• If you smoke, stop (and I mean *now*). Studies show that tobacco (and marijuana) negatively affects sperm count and motility.

• Drink alcohol only in moderation (red wine with dinner) or not at all. Heavy drinking (two to four alcoholic beverages per day) can interfere with sperm production.

• Strive for a healthy weight. Being too far above or below a healthy weight can cause hormonal disturbances that affect sperm counts and function.

• Take a nutritional supplement. Low levels of vitamins C and E and zinc negatively affect sperm. In fact, new research out of the Urology Institute at the Cleveland Clinic Foundation has found that vitamins C and E may help counteract abnormal amounts of free radicals, which may be responsible for infertility in some men.

• Avoid toxins such as pesticides, lead and other heavy metals. Lead is suspected to be the fifth leading cause of unexplained male infertility, according to a study published in *Human Reproduction.*

• Eat organically grown foods and drink plenty of water.

• Do not use steroids.

## Supplements for Male Infertility

*Vitamin C:* This vitamin and other antioxidants protect sperm from damage. If you smoke, it's very important to take vitamin C. Studies show that vitamin C reduces the clumping of sperm (agglutination), which can cause infertility. In fact, men with this condition who took 1,000 mg of vitamin C daily increased their fertility in one scientific study.

*Zinc:* Considered a fertility mineral, zinc impacts sperm count and impotence in men. In fact, infertile men are frequently low in zinc (contained in the semen). Some studies show that zinc supplementation (about 240 mg per day, an unusually high amount of zinc that should only be taken under doctor supervision) does indeed improve sperm count, not to mention the motility and physical characteristics of sperm. Taking 30 mg two times daily is customary. Keep in mind that long-term zinc supplementation may require adding 1–2 mg of copper per day to prevent copper deficiency.

*Arginine:* This amino acid is required for sperm production. A few studies show that L-arginine supplementation over a period of several months increases sperm count and structural quality (although if your sperm count is considerably low, the benefits are questionable). Infertile men with sperm counts greater than 10 million per milliliter may want to take up to 4 grams of L-arginine per day for several weeks and then have their count assessed again. L-carnitine, another amino acid, helps to normalize sperm motility in men with low sperm quality at a dose of 3 to 4 grams daily.

*Selenium:* This trace mineral has been tested in several studies, and in one double-blind trial of infertile men with reduced sperm motility, supplementation with selenium (100 mcg per day for three months) significantly increased sperm motility but did not impact sperm count. However, the stats are encouraging—11 percent of forty-six men receiving selenium achieved paternity anyway, compared with none of the eighteen men receiving a placebo.

*Vitamin B12:* Injections and oral supplementation of this vitamin can increase sperm counts. In one study, a group of infertile men were given oral vitamin B12 supplements (1,500 mcg per day of methylcobalamin) for two to thirteen months. Approximately 60 percent of those taking the supplement showed better sperm counts.

*Vitamin E:* A depletion of this vitamin can lead to infertility. When 100–200 IU of vitamin E were given daily to infertile couples (both partners), it led to a significant increase in fertility. Taking vitamin E also prevents free-radical damage that can destroy or impair sperm cells.

# Impotence: A Male Epidemic?

The Viagra phenomenon is one of the most dazzling success stories for the drug industry to date. This isn't surprising, considering that an estimated fifteen to thirty million American men are chronically impotent, and that figure is expected to rise as baby boomers enter their golden years. Approximately 25 percent of men over the age of fifty deal with impotence, and by the age of seventy-five, 55 percent of males will be affected. Despite these staggering percentages, impotence is not considered normal at any age.

Healthy men in their eighties and beyond can still function sexually, suggesting that a man's overall health status may be a more reliable predictor of impotence than age. Men who suffer from high blood pressure, heart disease or diabetes are up to four times more likely to become completely impotent later in their lives. Lifestyle factors such as smoking, alcohol consumption, inactivity, and the use of some medications also predispose men to sexual dysfunction. Narcotics, antihypertensive drugs, anti-anxiety medications, tranquilizers, and some antidepressants and diuretics can create temporary impotence. Over-the-counter antihistamines and decongestants have also been linked to transient impotence. In fact, over two hundred drugs list impotence as a possible side effect.

Up to 80 percent of erectile dysfunction (ED) cases are caused by physical factors, including obesity, low testosterone levels, arterial plaque deposits in the penis, low levels of good (HDL) cholesterol, hypothyroidism, chronic and nerve diseases, extreme fatigue and even lower back problems. (A small percentage of cases are also due to injury to or scar tissue in the penis.) These factors interfere with at least one of three things: penile nerve function, blood circulation to the penis, or proper stimulus from the brain.

# The Stress Connection to Erectile Dysfunction

I strongly believe that in the absence of physical factors, ED can be a manifestation of unmanaged stress. Unfortunately, most men who experience impotence fail to seek medical attention. Why? Because men typically associate impotence with notions of lost virility. Hence, the last thing they want to do is talk about it, even to a trusted family doctor who could offer them several treatment options—especially if stress is a problem.

Don't underestimate the role that stress or anxiety may be playing in cases of impotence. Emotional factors, workplace anxiety, strained relationships and the inability to relax can precipitate the problem. A study conducted with a group of men age forty to seventy concluded that after adjustment for age, a higher probability of impotence directly correlated with indexes of anger and depression. (It's important to keep in mind that while up to 80 percent of impotence is caused by physical factors, once an erection fails, psychological components kick in, compounding the problem.) Various studies suggest that anxiety is common among people with sexual dysfunction, emphasizing that anxiety management is crucial to normal sexual function and applies not only to men, but women as well.

Learning to relieve stress through relaxation exercises such as controlled breathing, massage, and the like can be very helpful. If you're not sure what kind of ED you have, you can purchase home impotence tests to determine whether the condition has a psychological or organic origin. These tests are set up prior to sleeping and determine if any erections occurred during sleep. If there are no erections while sleeping, organic factors are probably at work. If this is the case, contact a urologist for an exam. If you discover that erections do occur during sleep, but you still experience impotence when awake, then the problem may have a psychological basis and an appropriate counselor may provide solutions.

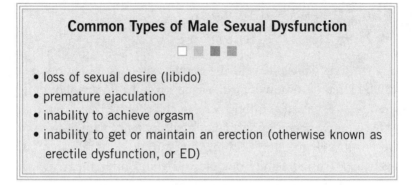

**Common Types of Male Sexual Dysfunction**

- loss of sexual desire (libido)
- premature ejaculation
- inability to achieve orgasm
- inability to get or maintain an erection (otherwise known as erectile dysfunction, or ED)

# Treating Erectile Dysfunction

Conventional treatment options for ED may include psychological and behavioral counseling. Get a complete physical to rule out the presence of cardiovascular disease or diabetes. A study reported in *JAMA* found that atherosclerosis of the main artery than runs through the penis is the primary cause of impotence in over half of men over the age of fifty. Drug treatments for ED include male hormone replacement therapy (testosterone, DHEA), sildenafil (Viagra), and medications inserted or injected into the penis (alprostadil). Penile vacuum devices and surgical options, such as penile implants and vascular repair, are usually considered last resorts.

While Viagra has enjoyed unprecedented popularity, more and more side effects continue to surface. Headaches and visual disturbances along with blackouts caused by sudden drops in blood pressure can occur, especially when Viagra is combined with nitroglycerine. According to the FDA's last update, there have been 123 deaths worldwide reported from March through July 1998 for patients taking sildenafil. Of the sixty-nine men who died in the United States, 74 percent had one or more risk factors for cardiovascular or cerebrovascular disease. In a recent article in the *Washington Post,* the FDA issued a warning to all doctors "that it may be too risky to give Viagra to whole groups of men including those who recently had heart attacks or very high blood pressure." Testosterone shots, other drugs and penile implants also come with health risks and significant side effects. In my opinion, it's far easier and safer to prevent erectile dysfunction. The best way to do that is with diet and exercise. As mentioned earlier in the chapter, regular exercise significantly lowers a man's risk for impotence, especially if he burns between 200 to 400 calories a day. The positive effects of exercise are even available to men who do not begin a regular routine until midlife. Exercise prevents impotence by keeping arteries open, which keeps a good flow of blood to the penis. Since impotence can be an early warning sign of heart disease, exercising early on may prevent it altogether by ensuring good cardiovascular health.

If you suffer from impotence, look at all aspects of your lifestyle and start from square one. Losing weight, exercising, reducing stress and eating a low-fat, high-fiber diet can help to improve circulation and counteract impotence caused by reduced blood flow. It's also important to avoid alcohol, tobacco and unnecessary medications, as well as limit your consumption of animal fats and highly sugared foods. Foods that are naturally high in zinc, essential fatty acids and important B vitamins are all crucial for good sexual function.

## Supplements for Sexual Dysfunction

*Vitamin E and Vitamin C with Bioflavonoids:* Vitamin E helps boost circulation and strengthen reproductive organs by effectively scavenging for dangerous free radicals. Because it helps to prevent arteriosclerosis, it may also prevent impotence. Vitamin E also works synergistically with vitamin C (especially when combined with bioflavonoids). Vitamin C helps maintain proper circulation and keeps the penile artery clean.

*Zinc:* This vitamin plays a profound role in maintaining healthy reproductive organs and contributes to normal prostate gland function. Zinc is involved in virtually every aspect of male reproduction, from keeping testosterone levels up to boosting sex drive. And because zinc is found in semen, it can easily become depleted. I like picolinate or gluconate varieties for maximum absorption. Keep in mind, however, that too much zinc can actually lower immune system function.

*DHEA (dehydroepiandrosterone):* This compound may improve sexual performance. In one double-blind trial, forty men with low DHEA levels who suffered from ED were given 50 mg of DHEA per day for six months. They experienced significant improvement in both erectile function and libido.

*Arginine:* This amino acid is necessary for the production of nitric oxide, necessary to achieve an erection. In one preliminary trial, men with ED were given 2,800 mg of arginine per day for two weeks. Six of the fifteen men in the trial improved, while none taking a placebo did. If your ED is prompted by impaired nitric oxide synthesis, arginine may offer an effective alternative to prescription drug medications.

*Asian ginseng (Panax ginseng):* This herb has been used for millennia as a sexual tonic for male potency. A double-blind trial found that 1,800 mg of Asian ginseng extract per day taken for three months helped improve libido and the ability to maintain an erection in men with ED. Another study found that a group of fifty men taking red ginseng experienced a 60 percent improvement rate in erectile dysfunction. The study stated that red ginseng was actually superior to trazodone, a prescription antidepressant drug used for certain kinds of impotence. Animal studies indicate that ginseng also raises sperm count and testosterone levels. It should also be noted that ginseng is especially effective for men over forty who suffer from any debilitating condition that frequently contributes to low sexual desire.

*Ginkgo biloba:* This brain-boosting herb may boost blood flow to the penis. One double-blind trial found improvement in men taking 240 mg per day of a standardized *Ginkgo biloba* extract for nine months. Another study of thirty men with drug-induced ED found that approximately 200 mg per day of *Ginkgo biloba* extract had a positive effect on sexual function in 76 percent of the men.

# Do Men Have a Feminine Side?

I can't let this chapter end without getting on my soapbox. After decades of working with and treating women, I've concluded that their ability to cope with pain and discomfort is nothing less than Herculean. Yes, this chapter addresses male health concerns, but take it from me, most men are clueless when it comes to the physical challenges faced by women. Can a man ever really empathize with a woman? My answer is no. There's a reason why males have lower pain thresholds than women—if we had to endure the physical and emotional trial of monthly bleeds, cramping and childbirth, we'd probably crumble. Furthermore, who among us can really imagine what it's like to find himself spread-eagle on a delivery table? I have a great deal of respect for the routine dehumanization and discomfort women typically endure as a result of the numerous gynecological tests and procedures.

Sadly, men have better access to quality medical care but unlike women, they don't take advantage of it. Furthermore, men (in general) appear to be less teachable when it comes to their health than women. Trying to get a man to change his eating habits and get off his duff is infinitely harder. Like I've said throughout the book, if you ignore your health, it will catch up to you.

The final, and equally important, point—men must acknowledge the emotional impact of their partner's hormonal makeup. Doing so can save countless hours of contention and resentment. Simply stated, don't take your wife or girl friend's cyclic behavior personally. A woman's cycle can significantly influence her emotions, her ability to cope, and her attitude toward family members. Believe me, the ebb and flow of estrogen/progesterone levels can make a woman want to put her fist through a wall. See the ups and downs for what they are. Listen to your partner, and learn to be supportive, not combative. Visiting a good ob/gyn together can also help.

# Glossary of Terms

*Acidification:* Using an acidifying agent (such as boric acid) to lower the pH of the vagina in order to fight yeast infections.

*Adenomyosis:* A type of endometriosis in which endometrial cells are present in the uterine wall that typically causes heavy periods and severe menstrual cramps.

*Adrenal androgens:* Male hormones produced by the adrenal gland which, when produced in excess, can lead to fertility problems in both men and women.

*Amenorrhea:* Refers to the complete absence of a menstrual period for six months or more in a premenopausal woman.

*Anovulation:* The failure to ovulate, which can be caused by hormonal imbalances or the use of oral contraceptives.

*Antibodies:* Protein molecules produced by the immune system to fight or attack foreign invaders. Autoimmune disease results when antibodies attack the body's own healthy molecules, cells or tissues.

*Antigen:* A substance that stimulates immune response.

*Antioxidant:* A substance that prevents damage caused by oxidation, which occurs naturally during metabolism and after exposure to toxins, injury, etc.

*Antiprostaglandin:* A compound that neutralizes problems (especially pain) caused by prostaglandin compounds.

*Artificial insemination:* The injection of semen into the vagina or uterus by means of a syringe or similar device.

*Bacterial vaginosis:* A bacterial vaginal infection that causes a burning sensation and a gray, malodorous discharge.

*Benign prostatic hyperplasia (BPH):* A condition occurring often in men over fifty where benign (noncancerous) nodules enlarge the prostate gland and tend to obstruct urination.

*Biopsy:* A diagnostic test used to rule out or confirm cancer. A tissue sample is removed and is examined under a microscope.

*Carcinoma:* A general term referring to a cancerous growth or tumor of epithelial origin (membranous cellular tissue that often protects other parts of the body).

*Carcinoma in situ (CIS):* A carcinoma in the stage of development when cancer cells are still in their site of origin and have not spread to other tissues.

*Cervical dysplasia:* Precancerous changes of the epithelial cells that cover the cervix and are usually detected by a Pap smear. They are often caused by HPV and may develop into cancer if not treated.

*Cervicitis:* An inflammatory condition of the cervix that can be caused by both infectious and noninfectious agents.

*Cervix:* The narrow lower or outer end of the uterus.

*Chemotherapy:* Generally refers to the use of very potent drugs or chemical agents to treat cancer.

*Colostrum:* A fluid produced by the breasts during the first days of lactation, containing essential nutrients and infection-fighting antibodies and other immune molecules called transfer factors.

*Colposcope:* A magnification instrument used to examine the cervix and vagina in women with abnormal Pap smears to detect cancer cells.

*Cone biopsy:* A surgical procedure that removes a cylindrical or cone-shaped piece of tissue from the cervix to diagnose cervical cancer.

*Contraceptives, oral:* A hormonal medication taken by mouth that prevents ovulation and pregnancy, and may also be used to treat PMS, irregular cycles and acne.

*Co-pay:* An arrangement where the insured pays a specified amount for various services, and the health carrier pays the remaining charges (i.e. the insured pays a ten-dollar co-pay per physician office visit rather than a percentage of the total cost).

*Corpus luteum:* A special group of endocrine cells that primarily produce progesterone immediately after ovulation.

*Corticosteroids:* Potent anti-inflammatory steroid hormones that are made naturally in the body or synthetically for use as drugs. The most commonly prescribed drug of this type is prednisone.

*Cortisol:* An adrenal-cortex hormone that is released during periods of stress and can negatively impact carbohydrate metabolism.

*Cryoablation:* Considered the safest form of endometrial ablation, this technique uses intense cold to destroy the uterine lining.

*Cryosurgery:* Using extreme cold (or freezing) to surgically remove abnormal tissue, such as in the cervix.

*Cryothalamotomy:* A surgical procedure used in the treatment of Parkinson's disease in which a supercooled probe is inserted into a part of the brain called the thalamus in order to stop tremors.

*D&C (dilation and curettage):* A procedure to scrape part or all of the endometrial lining of the uterus to treat abnormal uterine bleeding after menopause.

**Depo-Provera:** An artificial progestin administered by injection for contraceptive purposes.

**DES (diethylstilbestrol):** A nonsteroidal, synthetic estrogen used extensively from 1940–1971 for complications of pregnancy that was taken off the market because of serious side effects, including cancer and birth defects in the fetus.

**DHEA (dehydroepiandrosterone):** An androgen used by the body to make the sex hormones estrogen and testosterone that is now available in supplement form.

**Dihydrotestosterone:** The male hormone that can stimulate the growth of prostate gland cells and may be responsible for hair loss.

**Diosgenin:** A plant sterol derived from wild yam and soybeans that is considered a precursor to progesterone and is artificially converted to natural progesterone.

**Dysmenorrhea:** Refers to painful menstruation characterized by severe cramps, also often associated with heavy bleeding.

**Endometrial ablation:** A surgical procedure to destroy the uterine lining (endometrium), used to control heavy periods and related problems.

**Endometrial cancer:** A malignancy that occurs in the inner lining of the uterus (endometrium).

**Endometriosis:** A condition characterized by the presence of endometrial tissue in pelvic organs besides the uterus, especially the ovaries. It may cause pelvic pain and infertility.

**Endometrium:** The lining of the uterus.

**Erectile dysfunction (ED):** Also known as impotence, it is the inability to achieve and maintain penile erection. It can be caused by physical or psychological factors.

**Estradiol:** The most potent naturally occurring estrogen that is produced primarily in the ovaries and developing follicle and is primarily responsible for the formation of female sex characteristics.

**Estriol:** Another natural estrogen that is relatively weak. It is the main hormone secreted by the placenta during pregnancy.

*Estrogen:* Female sex hormone primarily produced in the ovaries, which stimulates female sex characteristics and promotes the growth and maintenance of the female reproductive cycle with progesterone.

*Estrogen excess (or dominance):* A term used when the normal balance of estrogen and progesterone is disrupted primarily because of inadequate progesterone production.

*Estrone:* One of three major estrogen hormones.

*Fallopian tubes:* Two hollow structures on either side of the uterus through which eggs travel to the uterus. Sperm typically fertilize the egg in the fallopian tube.

*Fertility treatment:* Any method or procedure used to enhance fertility or increase the likelihood of pregnancy through drug therapy or surgery.

*Fibromyalgia (FMS):* A syndrome of unknown cause characterized by muscular pain, fatigue and depression that primarily affects women.

*Free radical:* A molecule that has one or more unpaired electrons, making it highly reactive thereby destabilizing other molecules and causing serious tissue damage.

*Gatekeeper:* The primary care physician who must provide or authorize medical services for the member.

*Genistein:* The major isoflavone responsible for most of the beneficial effects of the isoflavone family.

*Gynecology:* The branch of medicine devoted to the treatment of women.

*HMO plan (health management organization):* A prepaid, restricted health plan designed to provide a complete network of medical service to plan members.

*Hormonal imbalance:* An umbrella term that is used to explain a myriad of women's health conditions.

*Hormone replacement therapy (HRT):* Typically refers to drug therapy using synthetic hormones to relieve symptoms associated with menopause. It now includes the use of natural hormone replacement products, with or without the use of synthetic hormones.

**Human papillomaviruses (HPV):** A number of viral strains that cause warts, particularly plantar and genital warts on the skin and mucous membranes. A number of these viruses are also linked to the development of cervical, anal, lung, head and neck cancers.

**Hysterectomy:** A term that refers to the surgical removal of the uterus. When ovaries and/or fallopian tubes are removed, the correct term is "salpingo-oophorectomy."

**Immune system:** The body's means of defending itself against injury or invasion by pathogens and foreign substances. It also rids the body of malignant or damaged cells.

**Impotence:** (see "Erectile dysfunction")

**Infertility:** The inability of a couple to conceive after one year of unprotected sexual intercourse.

**Insulin resistance:** A condition whereby cells become insensitive to the presence of insulin in the bloodstream, causing blood sugar levels to stay high.

**Integrative medicine:** A dynamic combination of different approaches to healthcare, including conventional, natural, alternative, complementary and herbal medicine.

**In vitro fertilization (IVF):** Fertilization of an egg performed in a laboratory, in a lab dish or test tube. Fertilized eggs may later be implanted in the uterus.

**Isoflavones:** Phytoestrogenic compounds that include biochanin A, formononetin, daidzein and genistein.

**Kegel exercises:** A series of exercises developed by Dr. Arnold Henry Kegel to strengthen pelvic floor muscles for controlling incontinence and enhancing sexual pleasure during intercourse.

**Laparoscope:** A small illuminated optical or fiberoptic telescope used during a laparoscopy to view internal organs.

**Laparoscopy:** A surgical procedure whereby a laparascope is inserted through a small incision to permit the viewing of organs in the abdominal cavity.

**Lupron:** The trade name for leuprolide acetate, a GNRH agonist primarily used to create temporary artificial menopause in women with endometriosis.

**Malignant melanoma:** One of the deadliest forms of skin cancer.

**Mammogram:** An x-ray image of the breast used to detect cancer.

**Managed care:** An approach to health care that focuses on the collaboration and coordination of medical services to avoid overlap and delays and to reduce costs. The patient receives only those medical services that are coordinated with their health care provider.

**Mastectomy:** The surgical removal of the breast or breast tissue and affected axillary (under arm) lymph nodes. There are several types of mastectomies including: simple, partial, total, modified radical and radical.

**Menorrhagia:** Heavy or prolonged menstrual flow.

**Micronized progesterone:** A prescription form of oral, natural progesterone that partially survives neutralization by the liver and is used by some physicians instead of natural progesterone cream.

**Natural progesterone cream:** A natural supplement consisting of USP progesterone that is applied topically and absorbed through the skin into the bloodstream.

**Needle aspiration:** A diagnostic test used to remove cells from a suspicious lump for microscopic analysis.

**Nurse practitioner (NP):** A registered nurse (RN) with advanced education and training that performs a variety of services with an emphasis on prevention and education.

**Obstetrical-gynecologist (ob-gyn):** A physician who specializes in the health maintenance and disease treatment of the female reproductive system, as well as pregnancy and childbirth.

**Olive oil, extra virgin:** The oil resulting from the first cold-pressed olives that is considered the healthiest and finest of the olive oils.

**Osteopenia:** Below-normal bone mass that can lead to osteoporosis.

**Osteoporosis:** A skeletal disease characterized by porous and brittle bones prone to fracture caused by the loss of calcium and other minerals.

**Ovarian cancer:** A malignancy that develops in one or both ovaries.

**Ovarian cysts:** Fluid-filled cystic structures similar to blisters that develop within the ovary and usually do not require treatment.

**Ovarian failure:** A condition characterized by an early cessation of menstruation that can occur in premenopausal women younger than forty years of age.

**Ovary:** One of a pair of female reproductive organs that produce eggs, as well as both estrogen and progesterone.

**Ovulation:** The release of a mature egg from the ovary that usually takes place in the middle of a woman's menstrual cycle.

**Ovum:** The egg or reproductive cell from the ovary also known as the female gamete that contains a woman's genetic information.

**Pap smear:** Introduced in 1943 by Dr. George Papanicolaou for whom it is named, the test is designed to detect the earliest stages of cervical cancer.

**Pelvic inflammatory disease (PID):** An infection of the reproductive tract that causes severe illness, high fever, and extreme lower abdominal pain. PID is the leading cause of infertility in women.

**Perinatology:** A sub-specialty of obstetrics concerned with perinatal care and the complications of pregnancy.

**Phytoestrogens:** Plant compounds with estrogen-like activity.

**PPO (preferred provider organization) plan:** An arrangement whereby an insurance company contracts with a group of medical care providers who furnish services at lower-than-usual fees in return for prompt payment and a certain volume of patients. PPOs are more flexible than HMOs because the insured can see health providers outside their provider's network for slightly higher out-of-pocket fees.

**Premarin:** A conjugated estrogen that is made from the urine of pregnant mares.

**Primary care physician:** A family practitioner/general practitioner, doctor of internal medicine, pediatric doctor, or gynecology doctor. HMOs require plan participants to select from an approved list of primary care physicians and access that physician first in order to receive approval for a specialist's care.

**Progesterone:** A female hormone secreted by the ovaries after ovulation takes place. Its primary role is to prepare the lining of the uterus for the implantation of a fertilized egg. Insufficient progesterone production may result in estrogen dominance.

**Progestins:** Synthetic compounds designed to mimic the actions of natural progesterone that are often combined with synthetic estrogen in HRT drugs and birth control pills.

**Prolactin:** A female hormone that stimulates milk production in lactating women and can be elevated when the thyroid is underactive. Elevated prolactin can prevent or decrease ovulation.

**Prostaglandin:** Any of a class of unsaturated fatty acids that are involved in the contraction of smooth muscle, the control of inflammation and the regulation of body temperature. They can also cause menstrual pain and discomfort.

**Prostate gland:** The male gland that produces the main constituent of semen.

**Provera (medroxyprogesterone acetate):** A synthetic derivative of progesterone used in injections or administered orally.

**Pruritus vulvae:** Localized or generalized itching of the vulva usually caused by contact dermatitis.

**Radiation therapy:** The use of high-energy X-rays, electron beams or radioactive isotopes to treat cancer. Radiation therapy has been shown to enhance the tumor-shrinking effects of chemotherapy.

**Rollerball ablation:** A method used to destroy the uterine lining by applying a ball-shaped, electrical probe directly to uterine tissue.

**Selective serotonin reuptake inhibitors (SSRIs):** A class of antidepressant drugs that sustain the presence of serotonin in the brain, thereby elevating mood.

**Serotonin:** A brain neurotransmitter which sustains mood and impacts hunger and behavior.

**Sonogram:** An image produced by an ultrasound, which uses high-frequency sound waves to create an image of internal organs, and to detect and monitor pregnancy.

**STD (sexually transmitted diseases):** A group of diseases transmitted primarily through sexual relations, i.e. HIV, HPV, chlamydia, herpes, gonorrhea, syphilis, etc.

**Testosterone:** The male sex hormone produced by the testes that stimulates and maintains the male reproductive system.

**Transfer factors:** Immune messenger molecules that are not species-specific and can transfer immune data from one mammal to another.

**Tubal ligation:** Surgical sterilization of a woman by obstructing or tying the fallopian tubes.

**USP progesterone:** Pharmaceutical quality progesterone. USP stands for "United States Pharmacopoeia," which is the international standard of purity for substances used in the manufacture of drugs and cosmetics.

**Uterine fibroid (leiomyoma uteri):** A generally round, benign growth of uterine muscle and connective tissue that rarely turns into cancer and is typically found in women with estrogen excess and may be hereditary.

**Uterine prolapse:** A condition that occurs when the supporting ligaments of the uterus give way, permitting the organ to drop from its normal position.

**Vaginal atrophy:** Shrinkage of tissue due to low estrogen levels in various areas including the vagina and pelvic floor, resulting in incontinence.

**Vaginal candidiasis:** An infection of the vagina caused by the overgrowth of the *Candida albicans* yeast.

**Vulva:** The external portion of the female genital tract.

**Wild yam root (*Dioscorea villosa*):** A plant native to Mexico that contains a compound called diosgenin, which is a known precursor to natural progesterone.

**Xenoestrogens:** Synthetic chemical substances that mimic estrogen and are primarily found in petrochemicals.

# Resources

## Patient Advocacy and HMOs

The Center for Patient Advocacy
www.patientadvocacy.org
1350 Beverly Road, Suite 108
McLean, VA 22101
(800) 846-7444
(703) 748-0402 fax
advocate@patientadvocacy.org

American Medical Association
www.ama-assn.org
515 North State St.,
Chicago, IL 60610
(312) 464-5000

Center for Health Care Rights
www.healthcarerights.org
520 S. Lafayette Park Place, Suite 214
Los Angeles, CA 90057
(213) 383-4519

Families USA Foundation
www.familiesusa.org
1334 G St. NW, Ste. 300
Washington, D.C. 20005
(202) 628-3030

National Committee for Quality Assurance
www.ncqa.org
2000 L St. NW, Ste. 500
Washington, D.C. 20036
(202) 955-3500
Webmaster@ncqa.org

## Dietary Supplements

www.vitaminretailer.com/SIE/articles/SpecialtySupplements

Nutrition Industry Executive
A-2 Brier Hill Court
East Brunswick, NJ 08816
(732) 432-9600
(732) 432-9288 fax

Food and Nutrition Information Center
www.nal.usda.gov/fnic/etext/000015.html

National Nutritional Foods Association
www.nnfa.org/services/science/gmp.htm
3931 MacArthur Blvd., Ste. 101
Newport Beach, CA 92660-3013
(949) 622-6272
(800) 966-6632
(949) 622-6266  fax
nnfa@nnfa.org

Food and Health Communications
www.foodandhealth.com/links/Nutrition/Supplements
/info@foodandhealth.com <info@foodandhealth.com

Center Watch Clinical Trials Testing Service
www.centerwatch.com/patient/patresrc.html
22 Thomson Place, 36T1
Boston, MA 02210-1212
(617) 856-5900
(617) 856-5901 fax

Dietary Supplement Information Bureau
Elliott Balbert, President
(818) 739-6000
ebalbert@natrol.com

National Library of Medicine
PubMed
www.ncbi.nlm.nih.gov/PubMed/
8600 Rockville Pike
Bethesda, MD 20894

## Women's Health

American Board of Obstetrics and Gynecology
www.abog.org/
2915 Vine Street
Dallas, TX 75204
(214) 871-1619
(214) 871-1943 fax
E-mail: info@abog.org

National Women's Health Information Center
www.4women.gov
8550 Arlington Blvd., Suite 300
Fairfax, VA 22031
(800) 994-WOMAN (1-800-994-9662) or
(888) 220-5446 for the hearing impaired

American College of Obstetricians and Gynecologists
www.acog.org
409 12th St., S.W., PO Box 96920
Washington, D.C. 20090-6920

Stanford University Medical Center
womenshealth.stanford.edu/advocacy.html
300 Pasteur Drive, Room HH333
Stanford, CA 94305-5317
(650) 723-7243
(650) 498-4320 fax
womenshealth@stanford.edu

Illinois State Medical Society
www.isms.org/patient/women.html
Women's Health Helpline @ 1-888-522-1282
Office of Women's Health Illinois Department of Public Health

National Women's Health Network
www.womenshealthnetwork.org
514 10th Street NW, Suite 400
Washington D.C. 20004
(202) 347-1140 (administrative)
(202) 347-1168 fax
(202) 628-7814 (health information)

American Medical Women's Association
www.amwa-doc.org/index.html
801 N. Fairfax Street, Suite 400
Alexandria, VA 22314
(703) 838-0500
(703) 549-3864 fax
info@amwa-doc.org

## Complementary Medicine

National Center for Complementary and Alternative Medicine
nccam.nih.gov
info@nccam.nih.gov

American Association for Health Freedom
www.apma.net/federalaffairs-natplan-text.htm
(800) 230-2762
(703) 759-0662
(703) 759-6711 fax
info@healthfreedom.net

Bastyr University
www.bastyr.edu
Pamela Snider, N.D. Associate Dean, Naturopathic Medicine
14500 Juanita Drive NE
Bothell, Washington 98011
(425) 602-3143
(425) 823-6222 fax
PSnider@bastyr.edu

Sheila Quinn, Executive Director
American Association of Naturopathic Physicians
www.naturopathic.org
601 Valley Street, Suite 105
Seattle, Washington 98109
(206) 298-0126
(206) 298-0129 fax
74701.3063@compuserve.com

Rosenthal Center for Alternative and Complementary Therapies
Columbia University, College of Physicians & Surgeons
www.rosenthal.hs.columbia.edu
630 W. 168th Street, Box 75
New York, NY 10032
(212) 342-0101
(212) 342-0100 fax

Dartmouth Biomedical Libraires
www.dartmouth.edu/~biomed/resources.htmld/altmed.htmld
www.dartmouth.edu/~biomed/resources.htmld/altmed.htmld
Hanover, New Hampshire 03755

Herbmed
www.herbmed.org

Ask Dr. Townsend
www.askdrtownsend.com

## Cancer

National Cancer Institute/Cancer.gov
www.cancer.gov/cancerinfo/treatment/cam

Office of Cancer Complementary Therapies
www3.cancer.gov/occam

BioImmune Inc.
breast.bioimmune.com/treatment/c_therapy/index.asp
8300 N. Hayden Rd. Suite A203
Scottsdale, AZ 85258
(480) 778-1618
(480) 778-1617 fax
(888) 663-8844

BreastCancer.Org
www.breastcancer.org/
PO Box 222
Narberth, PA 19072-0222
info@breastcancer.org

OncoLink
www.oncolink.com/about/article.cfm?id=1
University of Pennsylvania Cancer Center
3400 Spruce Street – 2 Donner
Philadelphia, PA 19104-4283
(215) 349-5445 fax

## Transfer Factor

4Life Reserach
www.4-life.com
850 South 300 West
Sandy, Utah 84070
(800) 851-7662 fax

## Nurse Practitioners

University of California San Francisco School of Nursing
nurseweb.ucsf.edu

National Organization of Nurse Practitioner Faculties
President, Diane Viens, DNSc, CFNP
1522 K Street, NW, Suite 702
Washington, D.C. 20005
(202) 289-8044
(202) 289-8046 fax
nonpf@nonpf.org

Nurse Practitioner Alternatives in Education, Inc.
4616 Old Dragon Path
Ellicott City, MD 21042
(410) 740-7078
(410) 740-7217 fax

California Association for Nurse Practitioners
2300 Bethards Drive, Suite K
Santa Rosa, CA 95405
(707) 575-8090
(707) 575-8620 fax
admin@canpweb.org

## Menopause

The Natural Health Website for Women
www.marilynglenville.com
health@marilynglenville.com

*Natural Alternatives to HRT: At Last a Breakthrough Approach to the Menopause and Osteoporosis That Could Dramatically Improve Your Health!* by Marilyn Glenville

## Natural Progesterone

*What Your Doctor May Not Tell You About Menopause: The Breakthrough Book on Natural Progesterone,* by John R. Lee

4Life Research
www.4-life.com
850 South 300 West
Sandy, Utah 84070
(800) 851-7662 fax

Pure Essence Laboratories, Inc.
P.O. Box 95397
Las Vegas, Nevada 89193
(888) 254-8000

## Disease Prevention

American College of Preventive Medicine
1307 New York Avenue, N.W., Suite 200
Washington, D.C. 20005
(202) 466-2044
(202) 466-2662 fax
info@acpm.org

PreventDisease.Com
www.preventdisease.com/home/contact.html
P.O.Box 2087, SQ1 Stn
100 City Centre Dr.
Mississauga, ONT, L5B 3C6, Canada
info@PreventDisease.com

American College of Preventive Medicine
1307 New York Avenue, N.W.  Suite 200
Washington, D.C. 20005
(202) 466-2044
(202) 466-2662 fax
info@acpm.org

# Bibliography

Adam, E., et al. "Vaginal and Cervical Cancers and Other Abnormalities Associated with Exposure *in utero* to Diethylstilbestrol and Related Synthetic Hormones." *Cancer Research.* 37, no. 4 (April 1977): 1249–1251.

Adlercreutz, H., et al. "Diet and Plasma Androgens in Postmenopausal Vegetarian and Omnivorous Women and Postmenopausal Women with Breast Cancer." *American Journal of Clinical Nutrition.* 49, no. 3 (March 1989): 433–442.

Adlercreutz, H., et al. "Diet and Urinary Estrogen Profile in Premenopausal Omnivorous and Vegetarian Women and in Premenopausal Women with Breast Cancer." *Journal of Steroid Biochemistry.* 34, no. 1–6 (1989): 527–530.

Adlercreutz, H., et al. "Excretion of the Lignans Enterolactone and Enterodiol and of Equol in Omnivorous and Vegetarian Postmenopausal Women and in Women with Breast Cancer." *Lancet.* 2, no. 8311 (11 December 1982): 1295–1299.

Agababian, Sandra. "Outsmarting Your HMO." *Health for Women. Woman's Day* Special Interests Publication. 8, no. 4 (fall/winter 1998): 82–83.

Agnusdei, D. and L. Bufalino. "Efficacy of Ipriflavone in Established Osteoporosis and Long-term Safety." *Calciferous Tissue International.* 61 (1997): S23–S27.

Albertazzi, P., et al. "Dietary Soy Supplementation and Phytoestrogen Levels." *Obstetrics and Gynecology.* 94 (1999): 229–231.

Albertazzi, P. "Purified Phytoestrogens in Postmenopausal Bone Health: Is There a Role for Genistein?" *Climacteric.* 5, no. 2 (June 2002): 190–196.

Albertazzi, P., et al. "The Effect of Dietary Soy Supplementation on Hot Flushes." *Obstetrics and Gynecology.* 91 (1998): 6–11.

Alhasan, S.A., O. Aranha and F.H. Sarkar. "Genistein Elicits Pleiotropic Molecular Effects on Head and Neck Cancer Cells." *Clinical Cancer Research.* 7, no. 12 (December 2001): 4174–4181.

Alvarez-Thull, L. and C.H. Kirkpatrick. "Profiles of Cytokine Production in Recipients of Transfer Factors." *Biotherapy.* 9, no. 1–3 (1996): 55–59.

Ambrosone, C.B., et al. "Breast Cancer Risk, Meat Consumption and N-acetyltransferase (NAT2) Genetic Polymorphisms." *International Journal of Cancer.* 75 (1998): 825–830.

Andersen, B.L., et al. "Stress and Immune Response after Surgical Treatment for Regional Breast Cancer." *Journal of the National Cancer Institute.* 90 (1998: 30–36.

Anderson, J.J., W.W. Ambrose and S.C. Garner. "Biphasic Effects of Genistein on Bone Tissue in the Ovariectomized, Lactating Rat Model. (44243)." *Experiments in Biological Medicine.* 217 (1998): 345–350.

Anderson, R. "The Immunostimulatory, Anti-inflammatory and Anti-allergic Properties of Ascorbate." *Advanced Nutrition Research.* 6 (1984): 19–45.

Armstrong, B. and R. Doll. "Environmental Factors and Cancer Incidence and Mortality in Different Countries, with Special Reference to Dietary Practices." *International Journal of Cancer.* 15 (1975): 617–631.

Armstrong, B.K., et al. "Diet and Reproductive Hormones: A Study of Vegetarian and Nonvegetarian Postmenopausal Women." *Journal of the National Cancer Institute.* 67 (1981): 761–767.

Ascherio, A. "Epidemiologic Studies on Dietary Fats and Coronary Heart Disease." *American Journal of Medicine.* 113, suppl. 9B (30 December 2002): 9–12.

Bagga, D., et al. "Effects of a Very Low Fat, High Fiber Diet on Serum Hormones and Menstrual Function." *Cancer.* 76 (1995): 2491–2496.

Baird, D.D., et al. "Dietary Intervention Study to Assess Estrogenicity of Dietary Soy among Postmenopausal Women." *Journal of Clinical Endocrinology and Metabolism.* 80 (1995): 1685–1690.

Barnes, A.B., et al. "Fertility after *in utero* Exposure to DES." *New England Journal of Medicine.* 303, no. 5 (31 July 1980): 280–281.

Barnes, S., T.G. Peterson TG and L. Coward. "Rationale for the Use of Genistein-containing Soy Matrices in Chemoprevention Trials for Breast and Prostate Cancer." *Journal of Cellular Biochemistry Supplemental.* 22 (1995): 181–187.

Barnes, S. "The Chemopreventive Properties of Soy Isoflavonoids in Animal Models of Breast Cancer." *Breast Cancer Research and Treatment.* 46 (1997): 169–179.

Barrett-Connor, E., et al. "The Postmenopausal Estrogen/Progestin Interventions Study: Primary Outcomes in Adherent Women." *Maturitas.* 27, no. 3 (July 1997): 261–274.

Barton, D.L., et al. "Prospective Evaluation of Vitamin E for Hot Flashes in Breast Cancer Survivors." *Journal of Clinical Oncology.* 16 (1998): 495–500.

Beisel, W.R. "Single Nutrients and Immunity." *American Journal of Clinical Nutrition.* 35 (1982): 417–468.

Betz, J.M., et al. "Chiral Gas Chromatographic Determination of Ephedrine-type Alkaloids in Dietary Supplements Containing Ma huang." *Journal of AOAC International.* 80, no. 2 (March–April 1997): 303–315.

Bonow, Robert, M.D. "Response to Heart and Estrogen-Progestin Replacement Study Follow-up (HERS II) published in July 3, 2002 *Journal of the American Medical Association (JAMA).*" Media advisory. American Heart Association. 9 July 2002.

Borradaile, N.M., et al. "Soya Phytoestrogens, Genistein and Daidzein, Reduce Apolipoprotein B Secretion from HepG2 Cells through Multiple Mechanisms." *Biochemistry Journal Immediate Publication.* (28 May 2002).

Borysov, V.A., et al. "The Adjuvant and Specific Activity of Transfer Factors to *Candida albicans.*" *Fiziologicheskii Zhurnal.* 44, no. 4 (1998): 3–9.

Boskey, E.R., et al. "Acid Production by Vaginal Flora *in vitro* Is Consistent with the Rate and Extent of Vaginal Acidification." *Infectious Immunology.* 67, no.10 (October 1999): 5170-5175.

Boucheix, C.L., et al. "Activity of Animal Transfer Factor in Man." *Lancet.* 1, no. 8004 (22 January 1977): 198-199.

Boyar, A.P., et al. "Response to a Diet Low in Total Fat in Women with Postmenopausal Breast Cancer: A Pilot Study." *Nutrition and Cancer.* 11 (1988): 93–99.

Boyd, N.F., et al. "Effects at Two Years of a Low-fat, High-carbohydrate Diet on Radiologic Features of the Breast: Results from a Randomized Trial." *Journal of the National Cancer Institute.* 89 (1997): 488–496.

Brezinski, A., et al. "Short-term Effects of Phytoestrogen-rich Diet on Postmenopausal Women." *Menopause.* 4 (1997): 89–94.

Brot, C., et al. "Relationships Between Bone Mineral Density, Serum Vitamin D Metabolites and Calcium: Phosphorus Intake in Healthy Perimenopausal Women." *Journal of Internal Medicine.* 245 (1999): 509–516.

Bulletti, C., et al. "Endometriosis: Absence of Recurrence in Patients after Endometrial Ablation." *Human Reproduction.* 17, no. 3 (March 2002): 844.

Burley, V.J. "Sugar Consumption and Human Cancer in Sites Other than the Digestive Tract." *European Journal of Cancer Prevention.* 7 (1998): 253–277.

"Cancer Group Tries to Link Fat, Cancer in Public Mind: 'Great American Weigh In' to Encourage Weight Loss." Associated Press. 19 February 2003. Available at www.cnn.com.

Carnes, Molly, M.D. "Health Care in the U.S.: Is There Evidence for Systematic Gender Bias?" *Wisconsin Medical Journal.* Guest Editorial. December 1999, 15–25.

Carpino, A., et al. "Low Seminal Zinc Bound to High Molecular Weight Proteins in Asthenozoospermic Patients: Evidence of Increased Sperm Zinc Content in Oligoasthenozoospermic Patients." *Human Reproduction.* 13 (1998): 111–114.

Cassidy, A., S. Bingham and K.D.R. Setchell. "Biological Effects of a Diet of Soy Protein Rich in Isoflavones on the Menstrual Cycle of Premenopausal Women." *American Journal of Clinical Nutrition.* 60 (1994): 333–340.

Challier, B., J.M. Perarnau and J.F. Viel. "Garlic, Onion and Cereal Fibre as Protective Factors for Breast Cancer: A French Case-control Study." *European Journal of Epidemiology.* 14 (1998): 737–747.

Chan, J.M., et al. "Dairy Products, Calcium, Phosphorus, Vitamin D, and Risk of Prostate Cancer." *Cancer Causes and Control.* 9 (1998): 559–566.

Chandra, R.K. "Nutrition and the Immune System: An Introduction." *American Journal of Clinical Nutrition.* 66, no. 2 (August 1997): 460S–463S.

Chapman, K.R., D.P. Tashkin and D.J. Pye. "Gender Bias in the Diagnosis of COPD." *Chest.* 119, no. 6 (June 2001): 1691–1695.

Chen, C.C., et al. "Adverse Life Events and Breast Cancer: Case-control Study." *British Medical Journal.* 311 (1995): 1527–1530.

Chen, F.P., N. Lee and Y.K. Soong. "Changes in the Lipoprotein Profile in Postmenopausal Women Receiving Hormone Replacement Therapy. Effects of Natural and Synthetic Progesterone." *Journal of Reproductive Medicine.* 43, no. 7 (July 1998): 568–574.

Chen, J., et al. "Effect of Oral Administration of High-dose Nitric Oxide Donor L-arginine in Men with Organic Erectile Dysfunction: Results of a Double-blind, Randomized Study." *British Journal of Urology.* 83 (1999): 269–273.

Chew, B.P. "Role of Carotenoids in the Immune Response." *Journal of Dairy Science.* 76 (1993): 2804–2811.

Chiechi, L.M. "Dietary Phytoestrogens in the Prevention of Long-term Postmenopausal Diseases." *International Journal of Gynaecology and Obstetrics.* 67, no. 1 (October 1999): 39–40.

Chow, R., J.E. Harrison and C. Notarius. "Effect of Two Randomised Exercise Programmes on Bone Mass of Healthy Postmenopausal Women." *British Medical Journal.* 295 (1987): 1441–1444.

Christy, C.J. "Vitamin E in Menopause: Preliminary Report of Experimental and Clinical Study." *American Journal of Obstetrics and Gynecology.* 50 (1945): 84.

Cohen, J.H., A.R. Kristal and J.L. Stanford. "Fruit and Vegetable Intakes and Prostate Cancer Risk." *Journal of the National Cancer Institute.* 92, no. 1 (2000): 61–68.

Collins, Karen Scott, M.D., M.P.H. "Midlife Women: Insurance Coverage and Access." *WREI Issue Brief.* Women's Research and Education Institute (WREI). May 2001. PDF.

Colston, K.W., U. Berger and R.C. Coombes. "Possible Role for Vitamin D in Controlling Breast Cancer Cell Proliferation." *Lancet.* I (1989): 188–191.

Condra, M., et al. "Prevalence and Significance of Tobacco Smoking in Impotence." *Urology.* 27 (1986): 495–498.

Cook, N.R., et al. "Beta-carotene Supplementation for Patients with Low Baseline Levels and Decreased Risks of Total and Prostate Carcinoma." *Cancer.* 86 (1999): 1783–1792.

Covens, A.L., P. Christopher and R.F. Casper. "The Effect of Dietary Supplementation with Fish Oil Fatty Acids on Surgically Induced Endometriosis in the Rabbit." *Fertility and Sterility.* 49 (1988): 698–703.

Cover, C.M., et al. "Indole-3-carbinol and Tamoxifen Cooperate to Arrest the Cell Cycle of MCF-7 Breast Cancer Cells." *Cancer Research.* 59 (1999): 1244–1251.

Czeizel, A.E., J. Metneki and I. Dudas. "The Effect of Preconceptional

Multivitamin Supplementation on Fertility." *International Journal of Vitamin and Nutrition Research.* 66 (1996): 55–58.

Dampier, K., et al. "Differences between Human Breast Cell Lines in Susceptibility towards Growth Inhibition by Genistein." *British Journal of Cancer.* 85, no. 4 (17 August 2001) Aug 17: 618-624.

Davis, J.N., et al. "Genistein-induced Upregulation of p21WAF1, Downregulation of Cyclin B, and Induction of Apoptosis in Prostate Cancer Cells." *Nutrition and Cancer.* 32 (1998): 123–131.

de la Fuente, M., et al. "Immune Function in Aged Women Is Improved by Ingestion of Vitamins C and E." *Canadian Journal of Physiological Pharmacology.* 76, no. 4 (April 1998): 373–380.

Dennis, L.K. "Meta-analysis for Combining Relative Risks of Alcohol Consumption and Prostate Cancer." *Prostate.* 42 (2000): 56–66.

DeNoon, Daniel. "U.S. Healthcare System Fails Many Women." *WebMD Medical News.* 8 May 2002.

Derby, C.A., et al. "Modifiable Risk Factors and Erectile Dysfunction: Can Lifestyle Changes Modify Risk?" *Urology.* 56, no. 2 (1 August 2000): 302–306.

de Roos, N.M., M.L. Bots and M.B. Katan. "Replacement of Dietary Saturated Fatty Acids by Trans Fatty Acids Lowers Serum Cholesterol and Impairs Endothelial Function in Healthy Men and Women." *Atherosclerosis, Thrombosis and Vascular Biology: Journal of the American Heart Association.* 21, no. 7 (July 2001): 1233–1237.

de Stefani, E., et al. "Meat Intake, Heterocyclic Amines, and Risk of Breast Cancer: A Case-control Study in Uruguay." *Cancer Epidemiological Biomarkers and Prevention.* 6 (1997): 573–581.

Dhurandhar, N.V. "Increased Adiposity in Animals due to a Human Virus." *International Journal of Obesity and Related Metabolic Disorders.* 8 (24 August 2000): 989-996.

Dimai, H.P., et al. "Daily Oral Magnesium Supplementation Suppresses Bone Turnover in Young Adult Males." *Journal of Clinical Endocrinology Metabolism.* 83 (1998): 2742–2748.

DiPaola, R.S., et al. "Clinical and Biologic Activity of an Estrogenic Herbal Combination (PC-SPES) in Prostate Cancer." *New England Journal of Medicine.* 339 (1998): 785–791.

Dixon, R.A. and D. Ferreira. "Genistein." *Phytochemistry.* 60, no. 3 (June 2002): 205–211.

Dixon-Shanies, D. and N. Shaikh. "Growth Inhibition of Human Breast Cancer Cells by Herbs and Phytoestrogens." *Oncology Reports.* 6, no. 6 (November–December 1999): 1383–1387.

Dobak, J.D., et al. "Endometrial Cryoablation with Ultrasound Visualization in Women Undergoing Hysterectomy." *Journal of the American Association of Gynecological Laparoscopy.* 7, no. 1 (February 2000): 89–93.

Dorant, E., P.A. van der Brandt and R.A. Goldbohm. "Allium Vegetable Consumption, Garlic Supplement Intake and Female Breast Carcinoma Incidence." *British Cancer Research Treatments.* 33 (1995): 163–170.

Dorgan, J.F., et al. "Effects of Dietary Fat and Fiber on Plasma and Urine Androgens and Estrogens in Men: A Controlled Feeding Study." *American Journal of Clinical Nutrition.* 64 (1996): 850–855.

Dumonde, D.C., et al. "Eleventh International Congress on Transfer Factors." *Journal of Interferon Cytokine Research.* 20, no. 4 (April 2000): 439–441.

"Effects of Hormone Therapy on Bone Mineral Density: Results from the Postmenopausal Estrogen/Progestin Interventions (PEPI) Trial." The Writing Group for the PEPI. *Journal of the American Medical Association (JAMA).* 276, no. 17 (6 November 1996): 1389–1396.

Eicholzer, M., et al. "Smoking, Plasma Vitamins C, E, Retinol, and Carotene, and Fatal Prostate Cancer: Seventeen-year Follow-up of the Prospective Basel Study." *Prostate.* 38 (1999): 189–198.

Ellis, F.R., S. Holesh and J.W. Ellis. "Incidence of Osteoporosis in Vegetarians and Omnivores." *American Journal of Clinical Nutrition.* 25 (1972): 555–558.

Enriori, P.J., et al. "Effect of Natural 'Micronized' Progesterone on the Chorionic Gonadotropin Concentrations in Cyst Fluids of Women with Gross Cystic Breast Disease." *Journal of Steroid Biochemistry and Molecular Biology.* 73, no. 1–2 (May 2000 May): 67–70.

Estrada-Parra, S., et al. "Comparative Study of Transfer Factor and Acyclovir in the Treatment of Herpes Zoster." *International Journal of Immunopharmacology.* 20, no. 10 (October 1998): 521–535.

*Facts about Postmenopausal Hormone Therapy.* U.S. Department of Health and Human Services. National Institutes of Health Publication. October 2002. PDF.

Famularo, G. "Infections, Atherosclerosis, and Coronary Heart Disease." *Annals of the Italian Medical Institute.* 15, no. 2 (April–June 2000): 144–155.

Fay, M.P., et al. "Effect of Different Types and Amounts of Fat on the Development of Mammary Tumors in Rodents: A Review." *Cancer Research.* 57 (1997): 3979–3988.

Fentiman, I.S., et al. "The Binding of Blood-borne Estrogens in Normal

Vegetarian and Omnivorous Women and the Risk of Breast Cancer." *Nutrition and Cancer.* 11, no. 2 (1988): 101–106.

Feskanich, D., et al. "Protein Consumption and Bone Fractures in Women." *American Journal of Epidemiology.* 143 (1996): 472–479.

Feskanich, D., et al. "Vitamin K Intake and Hip Fractures in Women: A Prospective Study." *American Journal of Clinical Nutrition* 69 (1999): 74–79.

Fitzpatrick, L.A., C. Pace and B. Wiita. "Comparison of Regimens Containing Oral Micronized Progesterone or Medroxyprogesterone Acetate on Quality of Life in Postmenopausal Women: A Cross-sectional Survey." *Journal of Women's Health Gender-Based Medicine.* 9 (2000): 381–387.

Fraga, C.G., et al. "Ascorbic Acid Protects against Endogenous Oxidative DNA Damage in Human Sperm." *Proceedings of the National Academy of Sciences.* 88 (1991): 11003–11006.

Fraker, P.J., et al. "The Dynamic Link between the Integrity of the Immune System and Zinc Status." *Journal of Nutrition.* 130, suppl. 5S (May 2000): 1399S–1406S. Review.

Frentzel-Beyme, R. and J. Chang-Claude. "Vegetarian Diets and Colon Cancer: The German Experience." *American Journal of Clinical Nutrition.* 59, suppl. 5 (May 1994): 1143–1152S.

Fritz, W.A., et al. "Dietary Genistein Down-regulates Androgen and Estrogen Receptor Expression in the Rat Prostate." *Molecular and Cellular Endocrinology.* 186, no. 1 (15 January 2002): 89–99.

Fujisawa, T., et al. "Randomized Controlled Trial of Transfer Factor Immunochemotherapy as an Adjunct to Surgical Treatment for Primary Adenocarcinoma of the Lung." *Japanese Journal of Surgery.* 14, no. 6 (1984): 452–458.

Gambacciani, M., et al. "Effects of Combined Low Dose of the Isoflavone Derivative Ipriflavone and Estrogen Replacement on Bone Mineral Density and Metabolism in Postmenopausal Women." *Maturitas.* 28 (1997): 75–81.

Gandini, S., et al. "Meta-analysis of Studies on Breast Cancer Risk and Diet: The Role of Fruit and Vegetable Consumption and the Intake of Associated Micronutrients." *European Journal of Cancer.* 36 (2000): 636–646.

Garg, A. "The Postmenopausal Estrogen/Progestin Interventions Trial." *Journal of the American Medical Association (JAMA).* 274, no. 21 (6 December 1995): 1675–1676.

Garland, M., et al. "Alcohol Consumption in Relation to Breast Cancer Risk in a Cohort of United States Women 25–42 Years of Age." *Cancer Epidemiological Biomarkers and Prevention.* 8 (1999): 1017–1021.

Garland, M., et al. "Antioxidant Micronutrients and Breast Cancer." *Journal of the American College of Nutrition.* 12, no. 4 (August 1993): 400–411.

Geinster, J.Y., et al. "Preliminary Report of Decreased Serum Magnesium in Postmenopausal Osteoporosis." *Magnesium.* 8 (1989): 106–109.

Geller, J., et al. "Genistein Inhibits the Growth of Human-Patient BPH and Prostate Cancer in Histoculture." *Prostate.* 34 (1998): 75–79.

"Gender Equity in Coverage of Prescription Drugs." Press release. The American College of Obstetricians and Gynecologists (ACOG). 12 June 2001.

Gennari, C., et al. "Effect of Ipriflavone—A Synthetic Derivative of Natural Isoflavones—On Bone Mass Loss in the Early Years after Menopause." *Menopause.* 5, no. 1 (1998): 9–15.

Gerber, M., et al. "Relationship between Vitamin E and Polyunsaturated Fatty Acids in Breast Cancer. Nutritional and metabolic aspects." *Cancer.* 64, no. 11 (1 December 1989): 2347–2353.

Geva, E., et al. "The Effect of Antioxidant Treatment on Human Spermatozoa and Fertilization Rate in an *in vitro* Fertilization Program." *Fertility and Sterility.* 66 (1996): 430–434.

Geyer, S. "Life Events Prior to Manifestation of Breast Cancer: A Limited Prospective Study Covering Eight Years before Diagnosis." *Journal of Psychosomatic Research.* 35 (1991): 355–363.

Giardina, E.G. "Heart Disease in Women." *International Journal of Fertility and Women's Medicine.* 45, no. 6 (November 2000): 350-357.

Giovannucci, E., et al. "A Prospective Study of Dietary Fat and Risk of Prostate Cancer." *Journal of National Cancer Institute.* 85, no. 19 (6 October 1993): 1571–1579.

Giovannucci, E., et al. "A Prospective Study of Tomato Products, Lycopene, and Prostate Cancer Risk." *Journal of the National Cancer Institute.* 94, no. 5 (6 March 2002): 391–398.

Giovannucci, E. "Tomatoes, Tomato-based Products, Lycopene, and Cancer: Review of the Epidemiologic Literature." *Journal of National Cancer Institute.* 91 (1999): 317–331.

Golden, B.R., et al. "The Effect of Dietary Fat and Fiber on Serum Estrogen Concentrations in Premenopausal Women under Controlled Dietary Conditions." *Cancer.* 74, suppl. 3 (1994): 1125–1131.

Goodman, Lawrence. "Transplants Save Lives: Why Are Women Being Denied?" *Self.* November 2002, 164–167, 189–191.

Goverde, H.J.M., et al. "Semen Quality and Frequency of Smoking and

Alcohol Consumption—An Explorative Study." *International Journal of Fertility.* 40 (1995): 135–138.

Gozan, H.A. "The Use of Vitamin E in Treatment of the Menopause." *New York State Journal of Medicine.* 52 (1952): 1289.

Grady, D., et al. "Cardiovascular Disease Outcomes during 6.8 Years of Hormone Therapy: Heart and Estrogen/Progestin Replacement Study Follow-up (HERS II)." *Journal of the American Medical Association (JAMA).* 288, no. 1 (3 July 2002): 49–57.

Grodstein, F., et al. "Relation of Female Infertility to Consumption of Caffeinated Beverages." *American Journal of Epidemiology.* 137 (1993): 1353–1360.

Guo, T.L., et al. "Genistein and Methoxychlor Modulate the Activity of Natural Killer Cells and the Expression of Phenotypic Markers by Thymocytes and Splenocytes in F0 and F1 Generations of Sprague-Dawley Rats." *Toxicology.* 172, no. 3 (2 April 2002): 205–215.

Guo, T.L., et al. "Genistein Modulates Immune Responses and Increases Host Resistance to B16F10 Tumor in Adult Female B6C3F1 Mice." *Journal of Nutrition.* 131, no. 12 (December 2001): 3251–3258.

Hanabayashi, T., A. Imai and T. Tamaya. "Effects of Ipriflavone and Estriol on Postmenopausal Osteoporotic Changes." *International Journal of Gynaecology and Obstetrics.* 51 (1995): 63–64.

Harel, Z., et al. "Supplementation with Omega-3 Polyunsaturated Fatty Acids in the Management of Dysmenorrhea in Adolescents." *American Journal of Obstetrics and Gynecology.* 174 (1996): 1335–1338.

Harris, S.S. and B. Dawson-Hughes. "Caffeine and Bone Loss in Healthy Postmenopausal Women." *American Journal of Clinical Nutrition.* 60 (1994): 573–578.

Hart, J.P., et al. "Circulating Vitamin K1 Levels in Fractured Neck of Femur." *Lancet.* 2, no. 8397 (4 August 1984): 283.

Harvei, S., et al. "Prediagnostic Level of Fatty Acids in Serum Phospholipids: Omega-3 and Omega-6 Fatty Acids and the Risk of Prostate Cancer." *International Journal of Cancer.* 71, no. 4 (16 May 1997): 545–551.

Head, K.A. "Ipriflavone: An Important Bone-building Isoflavone." *Alternative Medical Review.* 4, no. 1 (1999): 10–22.

*Health Care Access and Coverage for Women: Changing Times, Changing Issues?* The Commonwealth Fund on Women's Health. New York: November 1999.

Heinonen, O.P., et al. "Prostate Cancer and Supplementation with A-tocopherol and ß-carotene: Incidence and Mortality in a Controlled Trial." *Journal of National Cancer Institute.* 90 (1998): 440–446.

Helzlsouer, K.J., et al. "Prospective Study of Serum Micronutrients and Ovarian Cancer." *Journal of the National Cancer Institute.* 88 (1996): 32–37.

Hennen, William J. *Transfer Factor.* Woodland Publishing. Pleasant Grove, Utah: 1998.

Hilton, Lisette. "Women Express Concern about Quality of Care, Access and Costs in National Survey." 20 May 2002. Available at www.healthcarehub.com

Holmes, M.D., et al. "Association of Dietary Intake of Fat and Fatty Acids with Risk of Breast Cancer." *Journal of the American Medical Association.* 281 (1999): 914–920.

Hopper, J.L. and E. Seeman. "The Bone Density of Female Twins Discordant for Tobacco Use." *New England Journal of Medicine.* 330 (1994): 387–392.

Hruska, K.S., et al. "Environmental Factors in Infertility." *Journal of Obstetrics and Gynecology.* 43 (2000): 821–829.

Hulley, S., et al. "Noncardiovascular Disease Outcomes during 6.8 Years of Hormone Therapy: Heart and Estrogen/Progestin Replacement Study Follow-up (HERS II)." *Journal of the American Medical Association (JAMA).* 288, no. 1 (3 July 2002): 58–66.

Hunt, I.F., et al. "Bone Mineral Content in Postmenopausal Women: Comparison of Omnivores and Vegetarians." *American Journal of Clinical Nutrition.* 50 (1989): 517–523.

Hunter, D.J., et al. "A Prospective Study of the Intake of Vitamins C, E, and A and the Risk of Breast Cancer." *New England Journal of Medicine.* 329 (1993): 234–240.

"Irregular Periods in Young Women Could Be Warning Sign for Later Osteoporosis." Press release. National Institutes of Health. 29 May 2002.

Ivarsson, T., A.C. Spetz and M. Hammar. "Physical Exercise and Vasomotor Symptoms in Postmenopausal Women." *Mauritas.* 29 (1998): 139–146.

Jacobs, D.R. Jr., et al. "Whole-grain Intake and Cancer: An Expanded Review and Meta-analysis." *Nutrition and Cancer.* 30 (1998): 85–96.

Jin, Y., et al. "Inhibition of Scavenger Receptor A Expression Treated with PMA by the Inhibitor of Tyrosine Protein Kinase Genistein." *Sheng Wu Hua Xue Yu Sheng Wu Wu Li Xue Bao* (Shanghai). 33, no. 1 (2001): 142–146.

Johnson, J.A. and J.L. Bootman. "Drug-related Morbidity and Mortality." *Archives of Internal Medicine.* 155 (1995):1949–1956.

Jolliet, P., et al. "Plasma Coenzyme Q10 Concentrations in Breast Cancer: Prognosis and Therapeutic Consequences." *International Journal of*

*Clinical Pharmacology and Therapy.* 36, no. 9 (September 1998): 506–509.

Ju, Y.H., et al. "Dietary Genistein Negates the Inhibitory Effect of Tamoxifen on Growth of Estrogen-dependent Human Breast Cancer (MCF-7) Cells Implanted in Athymic Mice." *Cancer Research.* 62, no. 9 (1 May 2002): 2474–2477.

Ju, Y.H., et al. "Physiological Concentrations of Dietary Genistein Dose-dependently Stimulate Growth of Estrogen-dependent Human Breast Cancer (MCF-7) Tumors Implanted in Athymic Nude Mice." *Journal of Nutrition.* 131, no. 11 (November 2001): 2957–2962.

Kaizer, L., et al. "Fish Consumption and Breast Cancer Risk: An Ecological Study." *Nutrition and Cancer.* 12 (1989): 61–68.

Kameda, H., E.J. Small and D.M. Reese. "A Phase II Study of PC-SPES, an Herbal Compound, for the Treatment of Advanced Prostate Cancer (PCa)." *Proceedings of the American Society of Clinical Oncologists.* 18 (1999): 320a

Kang, J.L., et al. "Genistein Prevents Nuclear Factor-kappa B Activation and Acute Lung Injury Induced by Lipopolysaccharide." *American Journal of Respiratory Critical Care Medicine.* 164, no. 12 (December 2001): 2206–2212.

Kang, K.S., J.H. Che and Y.S. Lee. "Lack of Adverse Effects in the F1 Offspring Maternally Exposed to Genistein at Human Intake Dose Level." *Food Chemistry and Toxicology.* 40, no. 1 (January 2002): 43–51.

Kelley, D.S. and P.A. Daudu. "Fat Intake and Immune Response." *Progressive Food and Nutritional Science.* 17 (1993): 41–63.

Kidd, P.M. "The Use of Mushroom Glucans and Proteoglycans in Cancer Treatment." *Alternative Medical Review.* 5 (2000): 4–27.

Kim, S.H., D.J. Morton and E.L. Barrett-Connor. "Carbonated Beverage Consumption and Bone Mineral Density among Older Women: The Rancho Bernardo Study." *American Journal of Public Health.* 87 (1997):276–279.

Kimmick, G.G., R.A. Bell and R.M. Bostick. "Vitamin E and Breast Cancer: A Review." *Nutrition and Cancer.* 27 (1997): 109–117.

Kirkpatrick, C.H. "Activities and Characteristics of Transfer Factors." *Biotherapy* 9, no. 1–3 (1996): 13–16.

Kirkpatrick, C.H. "Biological Response Modifiers. Interferons, Interleukins, and Transfer Factor." *Annals of Allergy.* 62, no. 3 (1989): 170–176.

Kirkpatrick, C.H. "Structural Nature and Functions of Transfer Factors." *Annals of the New York Academy of Science.* 685 (23 June 1993): 362–368.

Kirkpatrick, C.H. "Therapeutic Potential of Transfer Factor." Editorial. *New England Journal of Medicine.* 303, no. 7 (1980): 390–391.

Kirkpatrick, C.H. "Transfer Factors: Identification of Conserved Sequences in Transfer Factor Molecules." *Molecular Medicine.* 6, no. 4 (April 2000): 332–341.

Knight, D.C. and J.A. Eden. "A Review of the Clinical Effects of Phytoestrogens." *Obstetrics and Gynecology.* 87, no. 5 pt. 2 (1996): 897–904.

Kojima, T., et al. "Hypolipidemic Action of the Soybean Isoflavones Genistein and Genistin in Glomerulonephritic Rats." *Lipids.* 37, no. 3 (March 2002): 261–265.

Krahnstoever Davidson, K. and L. Lipps Birch. "Obesigenic Families: Parents' Physical Activity and Dietary Intake Patterns Predict Girls' Risk of Overweight." *International Journal of Obesity and Related Metabolic Disorders.* 26, no. 9 (September 2002): 1186–1193.

Kris-Etherton, P.M. "AHA Science Advisory. Monounsaturated Fatty Acids and Risk of Cardiovascular Disease. American Heart Association Nutrition Committee." *Circulation.* 100, no. 11 (14 September 1999): 1253–1258.

Kristal, A.R., et al. "Vitamin and Mineral Supplement Use Is Associated with Reduced Risk of Prostate Cancer." *Cancer Epidemiology and Biomarkers of Prevention.* 8 (1999): 887–892.

Kruger, M.C., et al. "Calcium, Gamma-linolenic Acid and Eicosapentaenoic Acid Supplementation in Senile Osteoporosis." *Aging.* 10 (1998): 385–394.

Kumi-Diaka, J. "Chemosensitivity of Human Prostate Cancer Cells PC3 and LNCaP to Genistein Isoflavone and Beta-lapachone." *Biological Cell.* 94, no. 1 (February 2002): 37–44.

Kune, G.A. "Eating Fish Protects against Some Cancers: Epidemiological and Experimental Evidence for a Hypothesis." *Journal of Nutritional Medicine.* 1 (1990): 139–144.

Kynast-Gales, S.A. and L.K. Massey. "Effect of Caffeine on Circadian Excretion of Urinary Calcium and Magnesium." *Journal of the American College of Nutrition.* 13 (1994): 467–472.

La Vecchia, C., et al. "Fibers and Breast Cancer Risk." *Nutrition and Cancer.* 28 (1997): 264–269.

La Vecchia, C., et al. "Olive Oil, Other Dietary Fats, and the Risk of Breast Cancer." *Cancer Causes and Control.* (Italy) 6 (1995): 545–550.

Lamartiniere, C.A., et al. "Genistein Chemoprevention: Timing and Mechanisms of Action in Murine Mammary and Prostate." *Journal of Nutrition.* 132, no. 3 (March 2002): 552S–558S.

Laurenzana, E.M., et al. "Effect of Dietary Administration of Genistein,

Nonylphenol or Ethinyl Estradiol on Hepatic Testosterone Metabolism, Cytochrome P-450 Enzymes, and Estrogen Receptor Alpha Expression." *Food Chemistry and Toxicology.* 40, no. 1 (January 2002): 53–63.

Lee, J.R. "Osteoporosis Reversal: The Role of Progesterone." *International Clinical Nutrition Review.* 10 (1990): 384–391.

Le Marchand, L., et al. "Animal Fat Consumption and Prostate Cancer: A Prospective Study in Hawaii." *Epidemiology.* 5 (1994): 276–282.

Leonetti, H.B., S. Longo and J.M. Anasti. "Transdermal Progesterone Cream for Vasomotor Symptoms and Postmenopausal Bone Loss." *Obstetrics and Gynecology.* 94 (1999): 225–228.

Levy, J., et al. "Lycopene Is a More Potent Inhibitor of Human Cancer Cell Proliferation than Either A-carotene or ß-carotene." *Nutrition and Cancer.* 24 (1995): 257–266.

Levy, S.M., et al. "Perceived Social Support and Tumor Estrogen/Progesterone Receptor Status as Predictors of Natural Killer Cell Activity in Breast Cancer Patients." *Psychosomatic Medicine.* 52 (1990): 73–85.

Lewin, A. and H. Lavon. "The Effect of Coenzyme Q10 on Sperm Motility and Function." *Molecular Aspects of Medicine.* 18 Suppl. (1997): S213–S219.

Lian, Z., et al. "Preventive Effects of Isoflavones, Genistein and Daidzein, on Estradiol-17beta-related Endometrial Carcinogenesis in Mice." *Japanese Journal of Cancer Research.* 92, no. 7 (July 2001): 726–734.

Lloyd, T., et al. "Urinary Hormonal Concentrations and Spinal Bone Densities of Premenopausal Vegetarian and Nonvegetarian Women." *American Journal of Clinical Nutrition.* 54 (1991): 1005–1010.

Lockwood, K., et al. "Apparent Partial Remission of Breast Cancer in 'High Risk' Patients Supplemented with Nutritional Antioxidants, Essential Fatty Acids and Coenzyme Q10." *Molecular Aspects of Medicine.* 15 Suppl. (1994): S231–S240.

Lockwood, K., S. Moesgaard and K. Folkers. "Partial and Complete Regression of Breast Cancer in Patients in Relation to Dosage of Coenzyme Q10." *Biochemistry and Biophysical Research and Communication.* 199, no. 3 (30 March 1994): 1504–1508.

Malter, M., G. Schriever and U. Eilber. "Natural Killer Cells, Vitamins, and Other Blood Components of Vegetarian and Omnivorous Men." *Nutrition and Cancer.* 32 (1989): 271–278.

Mannan, M.T., et al. "Effect of Dietary Protein on Bone Loss in Elderly Men and Women: The Framingham Osteoporosis Study." *Journal of Bone Mineral Research.* 15 (2000): 2504–2512.

Marchigiano, G. "Calcium Intake in Midlife Women: One Step in Preventing Osteoporosis." *Orthopaedic Nursing.* 18, no. 5 (September–October 1999): 11–18.

Marcus, P.M., et al. "Physical Activity at Age 12 and Adult Breast Cancer Risk." *Cancer Causes and Control.* (United States) 10 (1999): 293–302.

Marsh, A.G., et al. "Bone Mineral Mass in Adult Lacto-ovo-vegetarian and Omnivorous Males." *American Journal of Clinical Nutrition.* 37 (1983): 453–456.

Martin-Du Pan, R.C. and D. Sakkas. "Is Antioxidant Therapy a Promising Strategy to Improve Human Reproduction? Are Antioxidants Useful in the Treatment of Male Infertility?" *Human Reproduction.* 13 (1998): 2984–2985.

Martin-Moreno, J.M., et al. "Dietary Fat, Olive Oil Intake and Breast Cancer Risk." *International Journal of Cancer.* 58 (1994): 774–780.

Medina, D. "Mechanisms of Selenium Inhibition of Tumorigenesis." *Advanced Experimental Medical Biology.* 206 (1986): 465–472.

Melchart, D. et al. "Immunomodulation with Echinacea—A Systematic Review of Controlled Clinical Trials." *Phytomedicine.* 1 (1994): 245–254.

Melchart, D. et al. "Results of Five Randomized Studies on the Immunomodulatory Activity of Preparations of Echinacea." *Journal of Alternative and Complementary Medicine.* 1 (1995): 145–60.

Melis, G.B., et al. "Ipriflavone and Low Doses of Estrogens in the Prevention of Bone Mineral Loss in Climacterium." *Bone Minerals.* 19, suppl. 1 (1992): S49–S56.

Mentor-Marcel, R., et al. "Genistein in the Diet Reduces the Incidence of Poorly Differentiated Prostatic Adenocarcinoma in Transgenic Mice (TRAMP)." *Cancer Research.* 61, no. 18 (15 September 2001): 6777–6782.

Mercuro, G., et al. "Effects of Acute Administration of Natural Progesterone on Peripheral Vascular Responsiveness in Healthy Postmenopausal Women." *American Journal of Cardiology.* 84, no. 2 (15 July 1999): 214–218.

Messina, M.J. "Legumes and Soybeans: Overview of Their Nutritional Profiles and Health Effects." *American Journal of Clinical Nutrition.* 70, suppl. 3 (September 1999): 439S–450S.

Messina, M.J., et al. "Soy Intake and Cancer Risk: A Review of the *in vitro* and *in vivo* Data." *Nutrition and Cancer.* 21 (1994): 113–131.

Meyer, F., et al. "Dietary Fat and Prostate Cancer Survival." *Cancer Causes and Control.* 10 (1999): 245–251.

Michnovicz, J.J. and H.L. Bradlow. "Altered Estrogen Metabolism and Excretion in Humans Following Consumption of Indole-3-carbinol." *Nutrition and Cancer.* 16 (1991): 59–66.

Mizunuma, H., et al. "Anticarcinogenic Effects of Isoflavones May Be Mediated by Genistein in Mouse Mammary Tumor Virus-induced Breast Cancer." *Oncology.* 62, no. 1 (2002): 78-84.

Nagata, C., et al. "Soy Product Intake and Hot Flashes in Japanese Women: Results from a Community-based Prospective Study." *American Journal of Epidemiology.* 153, no. 8 (15 April 2001): 790–793.

Nakajima, D., et al. "Suppressive Effects of Genistein Dosage and Resistance Exercise on Bone Loss in Ovariectomized Rats." *Journal of Physiology and Anthropology in Applied Human Science.* 20, no. 5 (September 2001): 285–291.

Neequaye, J., et al. "Specific Transfer Factor with Activity against Epstein-Barr Virus Reduces Late Relapse in Endemic Burkitt's Lymphoma." *Anticancer Research.* 10, no. 5A (1990): 1183–1187.

Neergaard, Lauren. "FDA Issues New Viagra Warnings." *The Washington Post.* 25 December 1998.

Nestel, P., et al. "Isoflavones from Red Clover Improve Systemic Arterial Compliance but Not Plasma Lipids in Menopausal Women." *Journal of Clinical Endocrinology Metabolism.* 84, no. 3 (March 1999): 895–898.

Netter, A., et al. "Effect of Zinc Administration on Plasma Testosterone, Dihydrotestosterone and Sperm Count." *Andrology.* 7 (1981): 69–73.

"New Facts about Estrogen/Progestin Hormone Therapy." Press release. The Women's Health Initiative (WHI). 9 July 2002. Available at www.nhlbi.nih.gov/whi.

Nieves, J.W., et al. "Calcium Potentiates the Effect of Estrogen and Calcitonin on Bone Mass: Review and Analysis." *American Journal of Clinical Nutrition.* 67 (1998): 18–24.

Norrish, A.E., et al. "Heterocyclic Amine Content of Cooked Meat and Risk of Prostate Cancer." *Journal of the National Cancer Institute.* 91 (1999): 2038–2044.

"N.Y. Sues Drug Firms over Incentives: Eliot Spitzer Targets Pharmacia, ClaxoSmithKline, Aventis." *Associated Press.* 14 February 2003. Available at www.msnbc.com.

O'brien, P.C., et al. "Vaginal Epithelial Changes in Young Women Enrolled in the National Cooperative Diethylstilbestrol Adenosis (DESAD) Project." *Obstetrics and Gynecology.* 53, no. 3 (March 1979): 300–308.

Oettgen, H.F., et al. "Effects of Dialyzable Transfer Factor in Patients with Breast Cancer." *Proceedings of the National Academy of Sciences.* 71, no. 6 (June 1974): 2319–2323.

Omu, A.E., H. Dashti and S. Al-Othman. "Treatment of Asthenozoospermia with Zinc Sulphate: Andrological, Immunological and Obstetric Outcome." *European Journal of Obstetrics and Gynecology and Reproductive Biology.* 79 (1998): 179–184.

Orenstein, Susan. "The Selling of Breast Cancer: Is Corporate America's Love Affair with a Disease that Kills 40,000 Women a Year Good Marketing–or Bad Medicine?" 2002. Available at www.business2.com/articles/mag/0,1640,46296,00.hmtl.

"Osteoporosis May Threaten Young Women." Press release. University of Arkansas. 31 July 2002.

Palkhivala, Alison. "Can Vitamin C or E Help Male Infertility?" *WebMD Medical News.* 22 June 2001.

Pandalai, P.K., et al. "The Effects of Omega-3 and Omega-6 Fatty Acids on *in vitro* Prostate Cancer Growth." *Anticancer Research* 16 (1996): 815–820.

Patisaul, H.B., et al. "Genistein Affects ER Beta- but Not ER Alpha-dependent Gene Expression in the Hypothalamus." *Endocrinology.* 143, no. 6 (June 2002): 2189–2197.

Peacock, S.L., et al. "Relation between Obesity and Breast Cancer in Young Women." *American Journal of Epidemiology.* 149 (1999): 339–346.

Pedrinaci, S., I. Algarra and F. Garrido. "Protein-bound Polysaccharide (PSK) Induces Cytotoxic Activity in the NKL Human Natural Killer Cell Line." *International Journal of Clinical Laboratory Research.* 29 (1999): 135–140.

Peinta, K.J. and P.S. Esper. "Is Dietary Fat a Risk Factor for Prostate Cancer?" *Journal of National Cancer Institute.* 85 (1993): 1538–1539.

Penn, N.D., et al. "The Effect of Dietary Supplementation with Vitamins A, C and E on Cell-mediated Immune Function in Elderly Long-stay Patients: A Randomized Controlled Trial." *Age and Aging.* 20 (1991): 169–174.

Persky, V.W., et al. "Hormone Levels in Vegetarian and Nonvegetarian Teenage Girls: Potential Implications for Breast Cancer Risk." *Cancer Research.* 52, no. 3 (1 February 1992): 578–583.

Peyser, Marc. "The Estrogen Dilemma." *Newsweek.* Special ed. Spring/Summer 1999, 35–37.

Pilewska, A. and A. Sendecka. "Cigarette Smoking as a Predicting Factor for Osteoporosis in Women." *Polski Merkuriusz Lekarski.* 10, no. 60 (June 2001): 414–415.

Pilotti, V., et al. "Transfer Factor as an Adjuvant to Non-Small Cell Lung Cancer." *Biotherapy.* 9, no. 1–3 (1996): 117–121.

Pizza, G., et al. "Effect of *In Vitro* Produced Transfer Factor on the Immune Response of Cancer Patients." *European Journal of Cancer.* 13 (1977): 917–923.

Potosky, A.L., et al. "Quality of Life Following Localized Prostate Cancer Treated Initially with Androgen Deprivation Therapy or No Therapy." *Journal of the National Cancer Institute.* 94, no. 6 (20 March 2002): 430–437.

Potter, S.M., et al. "Soy Protein and Isoflavones: Their Effects on Blood Lipids and Bone Density in Postmenopausal Women." *American Journal of Clinical Nutrition.* 68, suppl. 6 (December 1998): 1375S–1379S.

Prior, J.C., et al. "Conditioning Exercise Decreases Premenstrual Symptoms: A Prospective, Controlled 6-Month Trial." *Fertility and Sterility.* 47, no. 3 (March 1987): 402–408.

Prior, J.C. "Progesterone as a Bone-trophic Hormone." *Endocrinology Review.* 11 (1990): 386–398.

Pumford, S.L., et al. "Determination of the Isoflavonoids Genistein and Daidzein in Biological Samples by Gas Chromatography-mass Spectrometry." *Annals of Clinical Biochemistry.* 39, pt. 3 (May 2002): 281–292.

Purohit, V. "Moderate Alcohol Consumption and Estrogen Levels in Postmenopausal Women: A Review." *Alcohol Clinical Experience Research.* 22 (1998): 994–997.

Quinlan, D.J., D.E. Townsend and G.H. Johnson. "Safe and Cost-effective Laparoscopic Removal of Adnexal Masses." *Journal of the American Association of Gynecological Laparoscopy.* 4, no. 2 (February 1997): 215–218.

Raloff, J. "Reasons for Boning Up on Manganese." *Science News.* 27 September 1986, 199.

Rao, G.N., E. Ney and R.A. Herbert. "Influence of Diet on Mammary Cancer in Transgenic Mice Bearing an Oncogene Expressed in Mammary Tissue." *Breast Cancer Research and Treatment.* 45 (1997): 149–158.

Relea, P., et al. "Zinc, Biochemical Markers of Nutrition, and Type I Osteoporosis." *Age and Aging.* 24 (1995): 303–307.

Riby, J.E., et al. "Ligand-independent Activation of Estrogen Receptor Function by 3, 3'-Diindolylmethane in Human Breast Cancer Cells." *Biochemical Pharmacology.* 60 (2000): 167–177.

Richart, R.M., et al. "HPV DNA: Quicker Ways to Discern Viral Types." *Contemporary Obstetrics and Gynecology.* 33, no. 4 (April 1989): 112–124, 123–33.

Riis, B.J., et al. "The Effect of Percutaneous Estradiol and Natural Progesterone on Postmenopausal Bone Loss." *American Journal of Obstetrics and Gynecology.* 156 (1987): 61–65.

Rimm, E.B., et al. "Vitamin E Consumption and the Risk of Coronary Heart Disease in Men." *New England Journal of Medicine.* 328 (1993): 1450–1456.

Roberts, F.D., et al. "Self-reported Stress and Risk of Breast Cancer." *Cancer.* 77 (1996): 1089–1093.

Rohan, T.E., et al. "Dietary Folate Consumption and Breast Cancer Risk." *Journal of National Cancer Institute.* 92 (2000): 266–269.

Rolf, C., et al. "Antioxidant Treatment of Patients with Asthenozoospermia or Moderate Oligoasthenozoospermia with High-dose Vitamin C and Vitamin E: A Randomized, Placebo-controlled, Double-blind Study." *Human Reproduction.* 14 (1999): 1028–1033.

Rosano, G.M., et al. "Natural Progesterone Creams for Postmenopausal Women." *Drug Therapy Bulletin.* 39, no. 2 (February 2001): 10–11.

Rose, D.P. and J.M. Connolley. "Omega-3 Fatty Acids as Cancer Chemopreventive Agents." *Pharmacological Therapies.* 83 (1999): 217–244.

Rulm, L.A., et al. "The Effect of Calcium Citrate on Bone Density in the Early and Mid-Postmenopausal Period: A Randomized, Placebo-controlled Study." *American Journal of Therapies.* 6 (1999): 303–311.

Sahota, O. "Osteoporosis and the Role of Vitamin D and Calcium-vitamin D Deficiency, Vitamin D Insufficiency and Vitamin D Sufficiency." *Age and Aging.* 29 (2000): 301–304.

Salamone, L.M., et al. "Effect of a Lifestyle Intervention on Bone Mineral Density in Premenopausal Women: A Randomized Trial." *American Journal of Clinical Nutrition.* 70 (1999): 97–103.

Salonen, J., et al. "Risk of Cancer in Relation to Serum Concentrations of Selenium and Vitamins A and E; Matched Case-control Analysis of Prospective Data." *British Medical Journal.* 290 (1985): 417–420.

Schacter, A., J.A. Goldman and Z. Zukerman. "Treatment of Oligospermia with the Amino Acid Arginine." *Journal of Urology.* 110 (1973): 311–313.

Scheiber, M.D., et al. "Dietary Inclusion of Whole Soy Foods Results in Significant Reductions in Clinical Risk Factors for Osteoporosis and Cardiovascular Disease in Normal Postmenopausal Women." *Menopause.* 8, no. 5 (September–October 2001): 384–392.

Schulkind, M.L. and E.M. Ayoub. "Transfer Factor and Its Clinical Application." *Advanced Pediatrics.* 27 (1980): 89–115.

Schuurman, A.G., et al. "Animal Products, Calcium and Protein and Prostate Cancer Risk in the Netherlands Cohort Study." *British Journal of Cancer.* 80 (1999): 1107–1113.

Schuurman, A.G., et al. "Association of Energy and Fat Intake with Prostate

Carcinoma Risk: Results from the Netherlands Cohort Study." *Cancer.* 86 (1999): 1019–1027.

Scibona, M., et al. "L-arginine and Male Infertility." *Minerva Urology Nefrology.* 46 (1994): 251–253.

Scott, R., et al. "The Effect of Oral Selenium Supplementation on Human Sperm Motility." *British Journal of Urology.* 82 (1998): 76–80.

Shamberger, R.J., et al. "Antioxidants and Cancer. I. Selenium in the Blood of Normals and Cancer Patients." *Journal of the National Cancer Institute.* 4 (1973): 863–870.

Shangold, M.M. "Exercise in the Menopausal Woman." *Obstetrics and Gynecology.* 75, suppl. 4 (April 1990): 53S–58S; discussion 81S–83S.

Shantha, S., et al. "Natural Vaginal Progesterone Is Associated with Minimal Psychological Side Effects: A Preliminary Study." *Journal of Women's Health Gender Based Medicine.* 10, no. 10 (December 2001): 991–997.

Shao, Z., J. Wu and Z. Shen. "Genistein Exerts Multiple Suppressive Effects on Human Breast Carcinoma Cells." *Zhonghua Zhong Liu Za Zhi.* 22, no. 5 (September 2000): 362–365.

Shao, Z. and Z. Shen. "Mechanism of Growth Inhibition by Genistein of Human Breast Carcinoma." *Zhonghua Zhong Liu Za Zhi.* 21, no. 5 (September 1999): 325–328.

Shibayama, T., et al. "Neonatal Exposure to Genistein Reduces Expression of Estrogen Receptor Alpha and Androgen Receptor in Testes of Adult Mice." *Endocrinology Journal.* 48, no. 6 (December 2001): 655–663.

Simonsen, N.R., et al. "Tissue Stores of Individual Monounsaturated Fatty Acids and Breast Cancer: The EURAMIC Study." *American Journal of Clinical Nutrition.* 68 (1998): 134–141.

Sinatra, S.T. "Coenzyme Q10 Concentrations and Antioxidant Status in Tissues of Breast Cancer Patients." *Clinical Biochemistry.* 33, no. 4 (June 2000): 279–284.

Small, E.J., et al. "Prospective Trial of the Herbal Supplement PC-SPES in Patients with Progressive Prostate Cancer." *Journal of Clinical Oncology.* 18 (2000): 3595–3603.

Smith, C.J. "Non-hormonal Control of Vaso-motor Flushing in Menopausal Patients." *Chicago Medicine.* 67 (1964): 193–195.

Smith-Warner, S.A., et al. "Intake of Fruits and Vegetables and Risk of Breast Cancer. A Polled Analysis of Cohort Studies." *Journal of the American Medical Association.* 285 (2001): 769–776.

Sohn, M. and R. Sikora. "*Ginkgo biloba* Extract in the Therapy of Erectile Dysfunction." *Journal of Secondary Educational Therapy.* 17 (1991): 53–61.

Somjen, D., et al. "6-Carboxymethyl Genistein: A Novel Selective Oestrogen Receptor Modulator (SERM) with Unique, Differential Effects on the Vasculature, Bone and Uterus." *Journal of Endocrinology.* 173, no. 3 (June 2002): 415–427.

Squadrito, F., et al. "The Effect of the Phytoestrogen Genistein on Plasma Nitric Oxide Concentrations, Endothelin-1 Levels and Endothelium Dependent Vasodilation in Postmenopausal Women." *Atherosclerosis.* 163, no. 2 (August 2002): 339–347.

Stanton, C.K. and R.H. Gray. "Effects of Caffeine Consumption on Delayed Conception." *American Journal of Epidemiology.* 142 (1995): 1322–1329.

Steege, J.F. and J.A. Blumenthal. "The Effects of Aerobic Exercise on Premenstrual Symptoms in Middle-Aged Women: A Preliminary Study." *Journal of Psychosomatic Research.* 37, no. 2 (1993): 127–133.

Steele, R.W., et al. "Transfer Factor for the Prevention of Varicella-zoster Infection in Childhood Leukemia." *New England Journal of Medicine.* 303, no. 7 (14 August 1980): 355–359.

Sumbayev, V.V. "Genistein Effect on Xanthine Oxidase Activity." *Ukrainskii Biokhimicheskii Zhurnal.* 73, no. 4 (July–August 2001): 39–43.

Talamini, R., et al. "Nutrition, Social Factors and Prostatic Cancer in a Northern Italian Population." *British Journal of Cancer.* 53 (1986): 817–821.

Tanaka, T., et al. "Inhibitory Effects of Estrogenic Compounds, 4-Nonylphenol and Genistein, on 7,12-Dimethylbenz[a]anthracene-Induced Ovarian Carcinogenesis in Rats." *Ecotoxicology and Environmental Safety.* 52, no. 1 (May 2002): 38–45.

Tanos, V., et al. "Synergistic Inhibitory Effects of Genistein and Tamoxifen on Human Dysplastic and Malignant Epithelial Breast Cells *in vitro.*" *European Journal of Obstetrics and Gynecology and Reproductive Biology.* 102, no. 2 (10 May 2002): 188–194.

Tashiro, T., et al. "N-3 Versus n-6 Polyunsaturated Fatty Acids in Critical Illness." *Nutrition.* 14 (1998): 551–553.

Tavani, A., et al. "Coffee Consumption and the Risk of Breast Cancer." *European Journal of Cancer Prevention.* 7 (1998): 77–82.

Tham, D.M., C.D. Gardner and W.L. Haskell. "Clinical Review 97: Potential Health Benefits of Dietary Phytoestrogens." *Journal of Clinical Endocrinology and Metabolism.* 83 (1998): 2223–2235.

Thune, I., et al. "Physical Activity and the Risk of Breast Cancer." *New England Journal of Medicine.* 336 (1997): 1269–1275.

Townsend, D.E. "Correlation between Colposcopically Directed Biopsy and Loop Excision." *Gynecology Oncology.* 64, no. 1 (January 1997): 180–181.

Townsend, D.E. "DES *in utero*—Managing the Consequences." *Contemporary Obstetrics and Gynecology.* 5, no. 1 (January 1975): 103–132.

Townsend, D.E. "Management of Adenosis." *Journal of Reproductive Medicine.* 16, no. 6 (June 1976): 290.

Townsend, D.E., et al. "Post-ablation-tubal Sterilization Syndrome." *Obstetrics and Gynecology.* 82, no. 3 (September 1993): 422–424.

Trichopoulou, A., et al. "Consumption of Olive and Specific Food Groups in Relation to Breast Cancer Risk in Greece." *Journal of the National Cancer Institute.* 87 (1995): 110–116.

"Unpleasant Side Effects." *Associated Press.* 30 April 2002. Available at www.cbsnews.com.

van Loan, M. and N.L. Keim. "Influence of Cognitive Eating Restraint on Total-body Measure of Bone Mineral Density and Bone Mineral Content in Premenopausal Women Aged 18–45: A Cross-sectional Study." *American Journal of Clinical Nutrition.* 72, no. 3 (September 2000): 837–843.

van Zandt, Keith B., M.D. "Osteoporosis and Fractures." Letter to the Editor. *American Family Physician.* American Academy of Family Physicians. 15 February 2000.

Viereck, V., et al. "Phytoestrogen Genistein Stimulates the Production of Osteoprotegerin by Human Trabecular Osteoblasts." *Journal of Cellular Biochemistry.* 84, no. 4 (2002): 725–735.

Vincent, A., M. Ruan and L.A. Fitzpatrick. "Gender Differences in the Effect of Genistein on Vascular Smooth Muscle Cells: A Possible Cardioprotective Effect." *Journal of Gender Specific Medicine.* 4, no. 1 (2001): 28–34.

Viza, D., et al. "Orally Administered Specific Transfer Factor for the Treatment of Herpes Infections." *Lymphok Reviews.* 4 (1985): 27–30.

Viza, D., et al. "Specific Transfer Factor Protects Mice against Lethal Challenge with Herpes Simplex Virus." *Cellular Immunity.* 100 (1986): 555–562.

Walaszek, Z., et al. "D-glucaric Acid Content of Various Fruits and Vegetables and Cholesterol-lowering Effects of Dietary D-glucarate in the Rat." *Nutrition Research.* 16 (1996): 673–681.

Wang, S.L., et al. "A Study on Occupational Exposure to Petrochemicals and Smoking on Seminal Quality." *Journal of Andrology.* 22 (2001): 73–78.

Wang, S.Y., et al. "The Differential Inhibitory Effects of Genistein on the Growth of Cervical Cancer Cells *in vitro*." *Neoplasma.* 48, no. 3 (2001): 227–233.

Wardle, J., et al. "Food and Activity Preferences in Children of Lean and Obese Parents." *International Journal of Obesity and Related Metabolic Disorders.* 25, no. 7 (July 2001): 971–977.

Wattenberg, L.W. and W.D. Loub. "Inhibition of Polycyclic Aromatic Hydrocarbon-induced Neoplasia by Naturally Occurring Indoles." *Cancer Reviews.* 38 (1978): 1410–1413.

Webb, C.M., et al. "Natural Progesterone, but Not Medroxyprogesterone Acetate, Enhances the Beneficial Effect of Estrogen on Exercise-induced Myocardial Ischemia in Postmenopausal Women." *Journal of the American College of Cardiologists.* 36, no. 7 (December 2000): 2154–2159.

Weber, K.S., et al. "Dietary Soy-phytoestrogens Decrease Testosterone Levels and Prostate Weight without Altering LH, Prostate 5alpha-reductase or Testicular Steroidogenic Acute Regulatory Peptide Levels in Adult Male Sprague-Dawley Rats." *Journal of Endocrinology.* 170, no. 3 (September 2001): 591–599.

Weisburger, J.H. "Lifestyle, Health and Disease Prevention: The Underlying Mechanisms." *European Journal of Cancer Prevention.* 11, suppl. 2 (August 2002): S1–S7.

White, L.M., et al. "Pharmacokinetics and Cardiovascular Effects of Ma-huang *(Ephedra sinica)* in Normotensive Adults." *Journal of Clinical Pharmacology.* 37, no. 2 (February 1997): 116–122.

Whyte, R.I., et al. "Adjuvant Treatment Using Transfer Factor for Bronchogenic Carcinoma: Long-Term Follow-Up." *Annals of Thoracic Surgery.* 53, no. 3 (1992): 391–396.

Wietrzyk, J., et al. "Antiangiogenic and Antitumour Effects *in vivo* of Genistein Applied Alone or Combined with Cyclophosphamide." *Anticancer Research.* 21, no. 6A (November–December 2001): 3893–3896.

Williams, Dailey & O'Leary. "FDA Launches Hearings Today." *AOL news & PRNewswire.* 8 August 2000.

Win, W., et al. "Different Effects of Genistein and Resveratrol on Oxidative DNA Damage *in vitro.*" *Mutation Research.* 513, no. 1–2 (15 January 2002): 113–120.

*Women's Satisfaction with Primary Care: A New Measurement Effort from the PHS National Centers of Excellence in Women's Health.* Reprint. The Jacobs Institute of Women's Health. *Women's Health Issues.* 10, no. 1 (2000): 1–9.

Wu, A.H., et al. "Soy Intake and Risk of Breast Cancer in Asians and Asian Americans." *American Journal of Clinical Nutrition.* 68, suppl. 6 (December 1998): 1437S–1443S. Review.

Wu, A.H., et al. "Tofu and Risk of Breast Cancer in Asian-Americans." *Cancer Epidemiological Biomarkers and Prevention.* 5 (1996): 901–906.

Wu, J., et al. "Cooperative Effects of Exercise Training and Genistein Administration on Bone Mass in Ovariectomized Mice." *Journal of Bone Mineral Research.* 16, no. 10 (October 2001): 1829–1836.

"Wyeth Informs Physicians of WHI Findings: Company Reaffirms Role of Combination HRT in Menopausal Treatment." Press release. Wyeth. 9 July 2002. Available at www.prempro.com/study.html.

Yan C. and R. Han. "Protein Tyrosine Kinase Inhibitor Genistein Suppresses *in vitro* Invasion of HT1080 Human Fibrosarcoma Cells." *Zhonghua Zhong Liu Za Zhi.* 21, no. 3 (May 1999): 171–174.

Yano, Y. "Effect of Dietary Supplementation with Eicosapentaenoic Acid on Surgically Induced Endometriosis in the Rabbit." *Nippon Sanka Fujinka Gakkai Zasshi.* 44, no. 3 (March 1992): 282–288.

Yaqoob, P. "Monounsaturated Fats and Immune Function." *Proceedings of the Nutrition Society.* 57 (1998): 511–520.

Yarzebski, J., et al. "A Community-Wide Survey of Physician Practices and Attitudes Toward Cholesterol Management in Patients with Recent Acute Myocardial Infarction." *Archives of Internal Medicine.* 162, no. 7 (8 April 2002): 797–804.

Zamora, Dulce. "FDA Takes Close Look at Popular Weight-Loss Herb." *CBS Health Watch.* 9 August 2000.

Zhang, S., et al. "A Prospective Study of Folate Intake and the Risk of Breast Cancer." *Journal of the American Medical Association.* 281 (1999): 1632–1637.

# Index